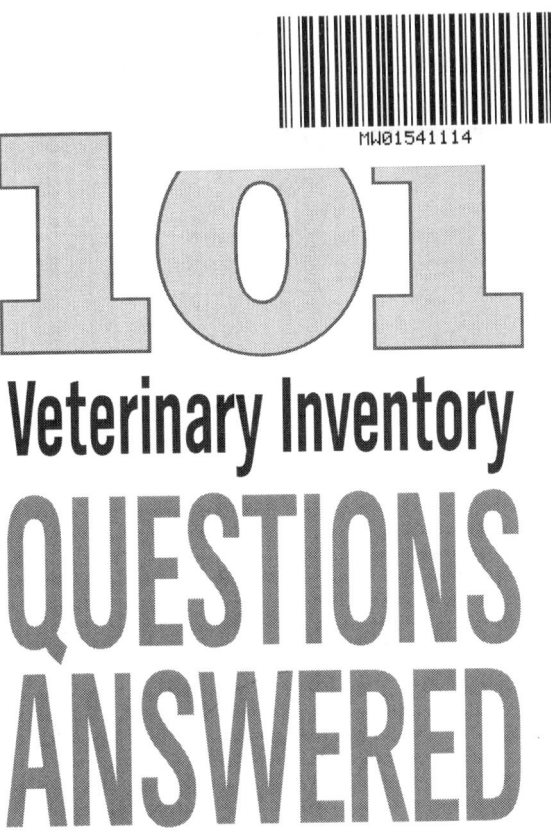

101 Veterinary Inventory QUESTIONS ANSWERED

James E. Guenther, DVM, MBA, MHA, CVPM, AVA

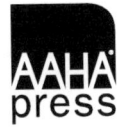

Veterinary Solutions Series
101 Veterinary Inventory Questions Answered
Copyright © 2010 by James E. Guenther

All rights reserved. No part of this publication may be reproduced or transmitted in any form or by any means, electronic or mechanical, including photocopying, without permission in writing from the publisher.

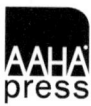
press

American Animal Hospital Association Press
12575 West Bayaud Avenue
Lakewood, Colorado 80228
800-252-2242 or 303-986-2800
press.aaha.org

Library of Congress Cataloging-in-Publication Data

Guenther, James E.
  101 veterinary inventory questions answered / James E. Guenther.
     p. ; cm.
  Other title: One hundred one veterinary inventory questions answered
  Other title: One hundred and one veterinary inventory questions answered
  Includes bibliographical references.
  ISBN 978-1-58326-126-2 (pbk. : alk. paper)
  1. Veterinary medicine—Inventory control. 2. Veterinary medicine—Equipment and supplies. I. American Animal Hospital Association. II. Title. III. Title: One hundred one veterinary inventory questions answered. IV. Title: One hundred and one veterinary inventory questions answered.
  [DNLM: 1. Practice Management—organization & administration. 2. Veterinary Medicine—organization & administration. 3. Equipment and Supplies—veterinary. 4. Hospitals, Animal. 5. Veterinary Drugs. SF 756.4]
  SF756.4.G84 2010
  636.089068'7—dc22
                                          2010031071

Printed in the United States of America

10 11 12 / 10 9 8 7 6 5 4 3 2 1

Book and series design by Erin Johnson Design

CONTENTS

Preface..v
Acknowledgments vii
   1. Efficient Ordering....................................1
   2. Training the Team..................................25
   3. Doctor Buy-In 41
   4. Benchmarks and Pricing..........................59
   5. Online Pharmacies 77
   6. Retail Centers and In-Hospital Use...................91
   7. Inventory Control.................................101
   8. Practice Management Software 121
   9. Controlled Substances and Injectables 137
   10. Inventory Manager Concerns 149
Resources..159
List of Contributors 161
About the Author 167

PREFACE

Inventory management is one of the most frequently forgotten or misunderstood aspects of running a veterinary practice. Veterinarians and practice managers have traditionally regarded inventory as something all practices need, but have given little thought to how to manage it *successfully*. The reason was simple: Inventory items were easier to sell than services.

To appreciate why inventory management is relatively new to the veterinary profession, consider the situation thirty years ago, when practices strived to reach a mythical success figure of $100,000 gross in a year. The idea was that, if a practice charged for its services appropriately and managed itself as a business, perhaps it could generate gross receipts of $100,000 or more. To achieve this goal took practice management skill, but inventory was not being managed because it was seen simply as a necessary portion of the practice that could manage itself.

In the early 1990s, veterinarians began to see once-a-month heartworm and flea products. Product sales of inventory items skyrocketed, thanks to an exclusive group of veterinary-only products that practices could sell. These products increased the gross revenue of practices tremendously, and consequently inventory was still not perceived as an important revenue source to be managed. Even when drug companies started to push practices to buy bulk quantities by offering discounts, veterinarians bought more of these products without understanding how bulk purchases could affect their cash flow.

In today's marketplace, veterinary practices are faced with competition for the consumer's dollar for products from online retailers, $3 and $4 generics, big-box pet stores, eBay, and other new businesses. Veterinarians realize they need to manage their practices as businesses, including all of their valuable assets: money, people, equipment, and yes, inventory too. But now that they are ready to

PREFACE

learn how to manage inventory, there are few sources of veterinary-specific information to give them the tools they need. This book was designed to fill that gap and help veterinary practices improve their inventory management in ways that will save them time and reduce hassles, protect the bottom line and cash flow, and allow them to better meet the needs of their clients.

AAHA Press sent out a survey to identify 101 common questions regarding inventory. The plan was to provide answers to these questions in the form of a practical, hands-on guide that was easy to use and apply. The answers presented here are a synthesis of the concerns and responses of in-the-trenches practice and inventory managers, aided by a consultant's perspective on how to make the most of inventory management and product sales.

Inventory is the buzzword for 21st-century veterinary practices and is one of the last frontiers for their success. These pages represent a major step forward in veterinary inventory management. With this tool, not only will your confidence as an inventory manager grow, but you will also tame the inventory monster.

ACKNOWLEDGMENTS

I would like to thank the many hardworking, dedicated veterinary professionals whose survey responses resulted in the wealth of insight and information in this book. These invaluable contributions have improved my knowledge, and I know you will find them to be equally helpful in improving and managing your practice's inventory system.

Special thanks go to Michelle Guercio, CVT, CVPM, for reviewing this book and offering many helpful suggestions. Also to Bess Maher for her support and continuous assistance with ensuring that all responses are easily understood.

CHAPTER 1: EFFICIENT ORDERING

How do I make the ordering process more efficient?

Inventory efficiency starts with a good inventory management system. Designate a smart, detail-oriented, cost-conscious, and assertive employee as the inventory manager. This person could be the practice manager or another staff member who demonstrates these traits. He or she should develop and implement protocols for managing inventory that are easy for staff to understand and follow. Among these protocols should be a system for ordering, one that the inventory manager has developed to fit the needs and style—the culture—of the practice.

One method of efficient ordering is to develop a "zone" system, in which several people are involved in managing areas or zones within the practice. Have the inventory manager develop a spreadsheet with a list of the products for each zone. This will enhance the process and make it easier for zone managers to count their products. On a weekly basis, zone managers perform an inventory count and enter their product counts in the spreadsheet, which is returned to the inventory manager for use in preparing purchase orders.

In an alternative method to the zone system, the inventory manager creates an order sheet and posts it so that staff can add products as needed. The sheet can be posted weekly, typically every Monday, and retrieved for preparing purchase orders a day later. The posting of a "need list" can be used in conjunction with the "red tag" system, in which a colored card, usually red, is used to indicate a product is at its reorder point. On the tag should be the following: name of the product, name of the vendor you last ordered from, reorder quantity, and package price of the previous order. The key is to tag a quantity of stock that will last until the reorder arrives.

With either of these methods, it is essential to enter products into the practice management software regularly and accurately,

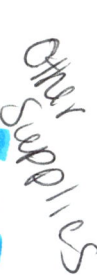

1

EFFICIENT ORDERING

both when they arrive and when they are used. Establishing reorder points within the computer system or via a spreadsheet allows for improved efficiency of ordering. With either method, reorder points can be reset to match seasonal needs for products. See Question 7 for information on setting reorder points.

In developing your preferred process, narrow your scope of ordering down to a few companies. The time it takes to do weekly price checks adds up quickly and can lower your profit margin. Consider performing price checks quarterly with your two or three preferred distributors on a select group of products. Look at the total cost provided by the distributor rather than at the cost of each individual product. Use this knowledge to help choose which vendors you will work with for the quarter.

Is price shopping multiple vendors really worth the time, or should we stick with just one or two vendors?

It is worth your time to check pricing with multiple vendors. Even though it is time-consuming to do so for every order, you should check on a quarterly basis. Quarterly price checking does not necessarily mean you will order from several vendors, but it should catch price increases before they become a problem and affect the practice's profitability.

By keeping your preferred list of vendors to just a few, you will save the time you usually spend searching for the best prices. You will also save money. Fewer phone calls or other forms of communication with vendors will reduce your ordering costs and staff time. Ordering costs can be tremendous when you are calling many places to save a dollar here and a dollar there. In some cases, ordering costs can be as high as 15 to 20 percent of the total unit cost.

Another plus to limiting your preferred list is the ability to create strong relationships with sales reps and inside order takers. Such relationships go a long way toward acquiring better pricing from vendors and improving pricing and inventory efficiencies for the practice. Cultivate vendor relationships by developing trust and establishing expectations with your vendors. By building bonds with vendors, you may get the best pricing without even asking.

When you have received good pricing on a product, ask the sales rep how you can lock in the price for a period of time. The vendor may require that you commit to ordering a certain quantity over a prescribed period of time. If this quantity is higher than what you need, see if one of your colleague practices could share in your order. Be creative when looking at your options.

Whatever pricing you get, always watch for mistakes in packing or invoices from vendors. Mistakes cost you time and money when you

EFFICIENT ORDERING

have to wait to receive the right product or must correct a billing error. A vendor's efficiency and follow-through may help in choosing which vendors to use. For instance, you may decide it is worth paying more for an item because a vendor is reliable and thorough.

➡ Do It Now

Start by listing your vendors by dollars spent. Next, evaluate your vendors by what they do for you on a regular basis—how good the relationships are and what is involved. Finally, rank them by which vendors are the most satisfactory.

EFFICIENT ORDERING

3

How many people should be involved in inventory ordering?

An ordering system will be more manageable if one person is the main inventory manager. The designation of one person—an inventory manager—to be in charge of ordering makes it easier to track and monitor pricing, sales, orders, back orders, specials, and returns. It also empowers the individual to enjoy a sense of ownership in managing the process and duties involved, which often directly results in improved efficiency of the inventory used and dispensed in the practice, as well as improved staff morale.

Even with one person assigned to do the ordering, it is always advisable to cross-train at least one other staff member to be a backup and perform the process when needed. Having a protocol in place is very helpful in training the backup person, as is having this person occasionally place an order to keep him or her familiar with the process.

It is wise to set up a series of checks and balances for all aspects of inventory management. Checks and balances are a means of ensuring that everyone, at every level of the process, is honest, and that everything ordered, used, and paid for is accounted for. They also represent a crucial component of what every inventory management system needs: a method to lessen the possibility of shrinkage (the loss of goods, especially through theft). If only one individual does all the ordering, unpacking, and data entry, error, or even shrinkage, is more likely to occur.

One way to implement this measure of inventory control is to have the inventory manager do all ordering because he or she is familiar with the process. But as shipments arrive, have a second person unpack and verify the order by comparing the packing slip with the purchase order.

EFFICIENT ORDERING

▶ Do It Now

Start by identifying, training, and empowering one key individual as the practice's inventory manager. Then develop a system for ordering, receiving, stocking, and entering data that allows for checks and balances at all levels of the process.

Order
unpack
Stocking
Enter Data

EFFICIENT ORDERING

[Handwritten margin notes: - Turn over 2 to 3 mos. - Exp - Returnable?]

4

How do we keep overhead low but still take advantage of multiple-purchase promotions?

Carefully evaluate all multiple-purchase promotions, recognizing that some will work, while others may not. Before entering into a commitment to accept a promotion, voice your concerns to the owners about keeping inventory low and do research to validate your concerns. Review usage and inventory turnovers of the product for your practice for the past 12 months. Then ask the sales rep or vendor to define the terms of the deal and demonstrate whether it actually will save the practice money. Now you can determine what the practice can afford to purchase based on cost savings, aiming for a minimum of 5 percent savings per month.

Ask yourself if the practice has the space for a larger than normal shipment of product without fear of shrinkage. If the practice ties up additional capital (money), make sure the product is in a secure, locked area with limited access. As a general rule, do not take advantage of any bulk-buying program that requires the practice to warehouse inventory that will not be turned over within two to three months.

Inquire about the dating of the product and whether the item can be returned for credit if it approaches its expiration date. These questions will help you make the final decision of whether or not to buy more than your usual quantity.

Remember that your pricing on promotions is a savings for the practice, not necessarily for the client. Even if you get a discount for the purchase, you should not automatically lower the selling price to your clients. Markups should be based on the cost of purchasing a nondiscounted quantity. Ultimately, the price difference improves the practice's profit margin.

[Handwritten note: Never decrease markup w/ discount]

EFFICIENT ORDERING

How can we accurately compare prices between vendors?

Your job is to shop for vendors that will provide outstanding service and give the practice great value for the price, just as clients do with your practice. Comparing prices on a weekly basis is counterproductive. In most cases, the differences in the total bill for these items will be pennies. Instead, it is a good idea to compare prices once per quarter for specific items, especially the prices of your "A" products (see Question 7).

When performing price comparisons, send a standardized list to vendors in the same manner, such as by fax or e-mail, to ensure that you are comparing "apples to apples." Track the time it takes for vendors to get back to you with their prices, and check for accuracy of the price estimate. Lower costs may be the deciding factor, but often price is not everything and you may have to look beyond price savings.

In cases when vendors quote similar prices, less tangible characteristics will be what bring a vendor to the top of your list. A few intangibles to consider are (1) vendor's accuracy and response time, (2) a strong relationship you or the owner have with the vendor, (3) free shipping offered by the vendor, and (4) if the vendor partners offer educational or consultative services in addition to sales. You will often be able to rely on one or two vendors for almost everything you order. After you decide on a vendor and agree to the quoted pricing, see if you can "lock in" those costs for the quarter.

⇒ **Do It Now**

Sit down at the computer and create a standard list of products you want to compare as a Microsoft Word document. This will become your template for checking prices from your vendors in the future.

EFFICIENT ORDERING   *Special Orders? 7 to 10 days*

How do I keep up with special orders—that is, products ordered for specific clients?

There are many ways to keep up with special orders. One way is to maintain a special-order board or basket dedicated to those requests. The requests are usually taken by a receptionist and sent to the inventory manager's attention via board or basket. When the product is ordered, make sure the order date is written on the purchase order, in case the client calls to ask whether it has been ordered. When the product arrives, call the client immediately. Remember to ask your special-order clients to give you 7 to 10 days' notice on orders. This ensures (1) that the product is on hand before the client runs out of a current supply, and (2) that additional shipping costs are not incurred when placing small orders.

Another way to keep up with special orders is to prepare a special-order form to be used for all special need products that clients request. The form should include client/patient information, space for the doctor's approval if approval is needed, date ordered, date received, and date the client was called about arrival of the product. Make sure that, upon arrival, all special-order products are clearly marked with the owners' names and placed in a "to be picked up" area. This will reduce the chances of the product being placed in the hospital central pharmacy and being used accidentally for the wrong patient. Be sure to have owners sign to confirm pickup.

Know your clients' histories. Special orders may be associated with additional expenses that should be passed on to the client. Determine if these are good clients who will pay for the product, or who will decide not to pick up the order when it arrives, leaving the practice with a product that may have to be returned and assessed a restocking fee. Strongly consider having all clients pay for a special-order product before you order it. This approach will lower

Pay ahead?

EFFICIENT ORDERING

the chances that the client will decide at the last minute not to pick up the product.

The key is to have a system in place for ordering, receiving, and dispensing special-order products. A special-order board, basket, or form are ways to track the progress of these orders. Also look for alternative ways to serve the client faster and better. For instance, ask another practice if it stocks the product, or use an online pharmacy. You never know what benefits might evolve from exploring alternatives for your clients and your practice.

EFFICIENT ORDERING

How do we determine the reorder point for a product?

Determining reorder points can be a simple task that involves basic math.

Step 1. The first step is to determine how much of the product you used in the previous year. Then add or subtract product based on your projections for the upcoming year. The "Report" function in your practice management software should feature product usage information. View the quantities used for the top 15 percent of your products (these are your "A" products) and make adjustments, if necessary, for this year.

> Quantity of product used in previous year ± projected quantity for upcoming year = quantity needed for upcoming year.

Step 2. Once you have identified the quantity needed for the upcoming year, the next step is to determine the daily usage of a product. First determine the approximate number of days you are open during the year. If you are open seven days a week, the number is 365. If you are open six days a week, it is 310 days. If you are open five days a week, it is 260 days. Then refer to your usage report and projected use for the current year. Let's say usage indicates that the quantity needed is 1,860 units, and that the practice will be open 310 days. The daily usage or demand is 1,860 divided by 310, or 6 units per day. Round up if you arrive at an average daily demand that is not a whole number.

> Anticipated quantity for upcoming year ÷ number of days the practice is open = average daily demand.

Step 3. Once you know the average daily demand for the product, you will need to determine the lead time it will take for the product

EFFICIENT ORDERING

to arrive at the practice. Lead time factors in the time it takes to process, order, and receive the product. Some practices, especially those that order only once a week, add a cushion of a couple days. Keep in mind that you are ordering enough to last you from when one order shipment arrives until the next shipment arrives. With lead time determined, the reorder point calculates as follows:

> Average daily demand × lead time = reorder point.

In our example, the average daily demand of 6 units is multiplied by a lead time of 3 days, which equals 18 units. That means the reorder point is when you have 18 units on the shelf. Place a reminder tag on the package with 17 units behind it, or enter 18 units into your computerized inventory module as the reorder point.

If you create a spreadsheet with the products that you decide need reorder points and enter all the above calculations, you have a template for future use.

Not all products will need reorder points. Be selective and apply the reorder point to the high-turnover or high-dollar-generating products, which are your "A" products: the products that generate the highest dollar amount.

You may have products that move more quickly than others at certain times of the year. To maintain your reorder points on those products, review your monthly usage reports from the year prior and add or subtract to determine the projected usage for the current year. Using the example above, if the average usage is 156 units per month (6 units per day × 26 days) but only 104 units are needed in December, the average daily usage becomes 4 units (104 ÷ 26). Lead time is still 3 days, but the new reorder point is 12 units.

➡ Do It Now

Start with heartworm preventives and determine your average daily demand for that product. From that calculation, determine your reorder point for heartworm preventives. That calculation can be your model for other order points.

EFFICIENT ORDERING

What is the most economical quantity to order at a time?

Once you determine a product's reorder point, based on the formula in Question 7, it is time to calculate order quantity. If you order too many units, product will sit on the shelf; if you order too few, you could run out of stock. By using the following economic order quantity (EOQ) equation, you can determine how much of a product to order (and reorder), while minimizing holding and personnel costs that can arise from placing orders.

$$EOQ = \sqrt{\frac{(2)(D)(O)}{(H)}}$$

In this equation, "D" is the product's annual demand, "O" is order placement costs (personnel) per order, and "H" is annual holding costs per unit ordered.

Using an equation with square roots may seem complicated initially, but financial calculators can perform this function with ease. If you are proficient in computer applications such as Excel or Numbers, the program can run the equation and automatically calculate the quantity for you.

Here's an example. If a product's annual demand is 1,860 units and the unit cost is $20, you have half of the information needed for the equation. The holding costs for most practices are 20 percent of the $20 unit cost, or $4, and the order placement cost is typically 10 percent of the unit cost, or $2. Now you have all of the necessary numbers to calculate the product's EOQ:

$$EOQ = \sqrt{\frac{2 \times 1{,}860 \times \$2}{\$4}}$$

EFFICIENT ORDERING

Or as follows:

$$EOQ = \sqrt{\frac{2(1{,}860 \times 2)}{4}}$$

This calculation gives you an EOQ of 43.13, which you would round to 43 units, to be ordered at any one time.

The EOQ equation determines the most cost-effective quantity to order based solely on the costs, which in turn allows you to effectively use data to optimize the profitability of your practice's inventory, ensuring both minimal operating costs and accuracy as part of your inventory model.

If you are new to EOQ, implementing it in your practice's inventory protocol can result in common mistakes, especially in determining the order and carrying costs. For instance, relying solely on benchmarks or published industry standards in the calculation, or factoring in too many costs associated with storage or handling fees, can lead to highly inflated costs. There will be some trial and error. Other factors, such as delayed billing (offered occasionally by vendors), discounts, and safety stock, can affect the quantities to order and must be carefully evaluated for accuracy.

Determining reorder quantities can also be accomplished by reviewing historical sales and usage reports to find the average 30-day supply needed for a specific product, which can be used as your reorder quantity. If you are deciding between ordering once a month or once weekly, a good compromise between the two is to order a two-week supply of a specific product twice a month. Doing so avoids having a large quantity of inventory on hand as a result of monthly ordering; it also prevents you from accruing personnel costs as a result of weekly ordering.

How often should items be evaluated and reorder points changed?

Reorder points should not be static. They should be evaluated on a regular basis and adjusted as needed. Reason for adjustment could be seasonality of the product, loss or gain in importance of the product with veterinarians, or a change in order frequency.

To properly evaluate the accuracy of your reorder points, review product usage reports monthly to determine whether products are moving from the shelves to the patient in the manner you anticipated. With the proper data, you will be able to identify trends of sales that can help set, or reset, reorder points for products. Ask vendors to provide you with the practice's buying reports, and compare these reports with your usage reports to gauge whether product selection and reorder points are in sync. Also, visually survey the practice's inventory weekly, ensuring that adequate quantities are on hand.

New product additions can be an experiment in arriving at reorder points. If the product is replacing another, use the outgoing product's reorder point until you develop a feel for or establish the frequency of usage. Be conservative with reorder points and adjust at least monthly until reaching an optimum quantity to have on hand.

The inventory manager should aim to continuously improve the product lines, turnover times, costs, and markups.

Product usage report
- are things moving off the shelves? quickly?

EFFICIENT ORDERING

10

How can we reduce our ordering to just once weekly?

It is not impossible to reduce ordering to once a week, but creating a system that works in your practice takes effort. The person selected for the job must be detail-oriented, cost-conscious, committed to accountability, prepared to create relationships with vendors and/or their representatives, and excited about the challenge of inventory control. Whether your practice uses a tag system, an inventory computer program, or zone counting, ultimate success comes by training everyone on the importance of inventory. It may take a while to move to weekly ordering, but as the system is refined, the time commitment decreases and managing inventory becomes more efficient and profitable. Here's how.

Start by understanding product usage for the practice by creating product usage and expiration reports from your practice management software. Develop reorder points and reorder quantities based on both actual and anticipated usage. Once the foundation of a system is in place, decide whether you will use the tag, computer, or zone system for your practice. There are pros and cons with all systems; what works well for a colleague's practice may not work for yours, and what worked for your practice yesterday may not work today.

Remember that educating everyone about the system is a challenge. Be patient and understanding with your staff as your practice moves to more efficient inventory management.

Once the system is in place, perform a "sight audit" of the inventory on a weekly basis. This is merely a way to ensure that the process is working. If you notice product shortages not accounted for on a purchase order, you can add the product immediately. This also helps you to notice where any breakdown in the system is occurring and plan to reacquaint the staff with the preferred method of managing inventory.

EFFICIENT ORDERING

Designing and implementing any system is a work in progress. There will be glitches—staff forgetting to remove the tags and put them in the common collection point, a missed charge that increases the quantity on hand in the computer, or zone managers not completing their counts on time. Be patient, be assertive, and reinforce the importance of inventory management to the staff whenever possible. For practices that have mastered once-a-week ordering, it required real energy, time, and effort by the entire practice team. A more realistic approach is to work toward a goal of ordering twice a week.

⇒ Do It Now

Develop your job description by defining the goals for the job. Then figure out how to accomplish those goals. Create a clear picture of how you will do this that includes methods to measure success.

Sight audit

11

I know I should use promotions for "A" products, but how much time should I spend pursuing distributors when looking for deals?

The cost of pursuing the best deal each time you need an "A" product (one of your top-selling products) will cost you more money, especially since most vendors today have similar prices for the same products. All products have indirect costs associated with them—the time you spend on ordering and storing each product.

Have you spent time creating great relationships with vendors? The best approach is to create strong relationships with two or three vendors from whom you order the bulk of your "A" products. This relationship will include your expectations on pricing, deals, freebies, and other matters; and it is based on the art of negotiation and letting each vendor know you have choices for ordering.

Several of your vendors probably handle most "A" products. Most vendors know the prices offered by other vendors and will offer competitive prices. If you have strong relationships with vendors, you have the best chance to get the best overall value for your dollar. Do not merely compare one product from two vendors—look at the total cost of the order. Sometimes one vendor will be higher or lower on certain items, but the total cost of an order will save you money.

On an annual basis, present your shopping list of "A" products to the vendors and see who has the best price for the total product list. See whether you can lock in prices for a specific period of time, with the understanding that you will order X amount during this period. Deciding the quantity to be ordered derives from your sales and/or usage reports for the same period last year and your budget predictions for this year (see Questions 7 and 8).

Negotiate price with your vendors, especially the ones with whom you have cultivated great relationships. They want your business as much as you want good pricing. By investing the time in building strong, lasting relationships, you will get a lot more value for your dollar than if you simply seek the best price.

Build Relationships

12

In our practice, we order as needed, sometimes three or four times per week. Is it more common to order on set days of the week, perhaps once or twice per week?

In general, the most cost-effective system is to order once or twice a week on specified days. This approach ensures that shipments arrive the same week they are ordered, and that you avoid incurring the soft costs of ordering too frequently, or as the need arises, which can be counterproductive to controlling inventory costs. In order to establish an optimal order frequency in your practice, you must set up good reorder points and reorder quantities based on usage and lead time.

Start by tracking the use of products by examining the usage report from the practice management software. This will assist in establishing reorder points for products. For more information on setting reorder points, see Questions 7 and 8. To determine reorder quantities, start with having approximately a month's supply on hand. Then fine-tune your reorder quantities from there.

Another factor to consider is the lead time needed for a shipment to arrive. In some locales, you can order and receive a product on the same day; in other areas, it may take several days for a shipment to arrive. Delivery issues play into establishing reorder points for products and can also help you determine the best days to place orders, ensuring delivery is the same week as ordered.

Some vendors may be exclusive distributors for certain products, such as diets. These vendors have established routes for delivering diets to certain areas on certain days. This can factor into the reorder points you establish for these specific products and on which days you order.

As you can see, this is not as simple as saying, "Mondays and/or Wednesday are the days I will order." Understanding your program

EFFICIENT ORDERING

and how you can make it the most efficient for the practice will make the difference. It will take time and energy to develop the plan that works best.

EFFICIENT ORDERING

13

How can we deter zealous sales reps?

It's tempting to think you can always just say no to zealous sales reps and not meet with them, but that might mean losing out on opportunities to save money on products your practice needs. Instead, consider setting specific days and hours when someone will speak with sales reps. It can actually help to spend quality time with a sales rep to discuss your expectations. Set the ground rules early, as you do with your staff. If sales reps know and understand your expectations, it will be easier to work with them.

Some sales reps are excellent because they are in the business of keeping their clients informed about meeting, products, and other opportunities. They know that if they create a lasting bond with you and your practice, the relationship may bring them many orders over time. Conversely, there are reps whose approach ensures that they most likely never will become preferred vendors. Take the time to analyze the sales force who calls on your practice. Establish criteria for your practice and create a list of preferred vendors and sales reps based on these criteria.

Consider asking an overzealous rep to schedule an appointment with you and the practice owner at which the rep pays for your time or provides a free product sample to try. If your business is worth it, the sales rep should be willing to pay for the appointment. Offering the "alternative" of not seeing them at all may get their attention. This approach may not suit your communication style, but it does allow for a dialogue that in the long term may be in the best interest of the practice.

Sales reps must understand and respect the ground rules that you and the owner establish for vendor communications if they want your business. Overzealous reps have to earn your trust. If a rep continues to be too assertive or unprofessional in attempting to

EFFICIENT ORDERING

gain your business, consider calling the company's sales manager and lodging a formal complaint. Sales reps and managers have performance reviews, and their supervisors need information to help with those evaluations.

Do not just sit back and keep quiet about the situation. That helps no one. If a client were a problem, you probably would "fire" him or her as a client. The same holds true for a sales rep. Be assertive, be firm, and take action *now*.

CHAPTER 2: TRAINING THE TEAM

14

How can we make our staff understand the need for efficient inventory management?

Staff members are not mind readers and tend to follow the actions of the leader—in this case, the practice owner or manager. Three issues are vital to the success of inventory management. First, management has to stress the importance of how inventory management relates to the bottom line and the profitability of the practice. Second, everyone in the clinic must be assigned an inventory expectation as a factor in performance reviews. Third, the staff should see the financials regarding inventory so they can understand the relationship of inventory control to their own interests: that better cash flow can result in better benefits and salaries.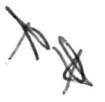

Management, especially owners, must emphasize and demonstrate a commitment to inventory control. If an owner or practice manager claims to believe in inventory control, but turns around and takes product from the shelves for personal use without paying for it, then that owner or manager is not demonstrating a belief in inventory control. The leader of the practice must "walk the talk" or else any communication with the staff has no meaning.

To make inventory management a part of staff performance evaluations, include items that assess inventory management behavior, such as questions that ask whether they are "careful and economical in handling supplies and equipment: unusually neat, clean, and orderly" or "careless, wasteful, disorderly, and untidy with equipment and supplies." Use questions that are aimed at making sure the staff understands and respects the economics associated with inventory items.

You might want to use an open-book management system to demonstrate the numbers associated with inventory. These can range from the amount of money "sitting on the shelves" to how much the practice loses on a regular basis because of shrinkage. Engage the staff and reward them for helping reduce loss. Explain how loss affects them. The more they understand about costs and waste, the sooner they will understand why controlling inventory is important for the patient, client, and practice.

Use staff meetings to emphasize the importance of inventory control. Explain that it takes selling three more of a product to recoup the monies from losing or not charging for just one item. You can be creative in demonstrating the importance of inventory control: Track the use of an in-house product, such as catheters, and have the staff guess how much was lost because one patient was not charged for use of extra catheters; reward the staffer who comes closest to the actual amount with a prize.

Finally, fix problems in the system. Create safeguards or checks and balances to improve inventory control, which will improve the profitability of the practice at the same time.

15

How can I train staff members to become aware of inventory needs and relay that information to me?

Train, train, and train some more: That is the best way to keep staff on top of the issue of inventory. Staff members can become frustrated when the practice runs out of products, so train them to prevent that from happening. Explain how their actions affect reorder information, turnover, and unhappy clients.

Training new staff members by having them shadow experienced staff members may help get the message across of what you expect from employees. This ensures that the newer staff member is educated about the importance of properly maintaining the clinic's inventory.

Part of training involves making sure there is a good inventory system in place. Explain how each area of the clinic keeps a certain number of inventory items. For instance, shelves are marked with the product name for ease of identification and there is a whiteboard or want list on which to post any items low in stock or missing. Teach staff that the person who uses the last of any item is responsible for recording it on the whiteboard or order list, if your practice uses this system (see Question 1).

Many items can be restocked from a central storage area, but staff must record any items they remove from central storage so quantities on hand can be adjusted for reordering purposes.

Regularly scheduled meetings are a great opportunity to train the entire staff on how to maintain inventory so the practice does not run out of items. This may not be a regular monthly portion of the client service meeting, but it surely could—perhaps should—be. Inventory is a huge expense in all practices. The staff needs to be aware of this and of how to avoid the pitfalls of shrinkage.

Consider asking management to implement some form of bonus

system for improving turnovers on products, not running out of product, or reducing shrinkage. Be creative in making inventory a priority for all staff members, since not having a good inventory system can affect the quality of medical care provided by your practice.

Finally, as an owner, practice manager, or inventory manager, lead by example and let staff know that the practice expects everyone to follow the lead of those who are managing inventory. Ultimately, it is not just the inventory manger's responsibility to control inventory; it is every staff member's responsibility.

16

How can we inform co-workers of losses so they can help improve inventory management?

Keeping co-workers informed about losses is vital. On a random monthly basis, select items to verify quantity actually on hand against the amount your inventory module says you should have on hand. If there is shrinkage, record it, and tell the staff the actual cost of the missing product and the corresponding loss of revenue for the practice. This will remind the staff what losses mean to the profit margin of the practice: less money for profit-sharing, raises, or new equipment.

At staff meetings, have an open discussion regarding the importance of inventory for the practice's patients, the clients, and the hospital. This can be presented as an exercise in examining the shrinkage of certain products and relating the cost of the product to the lost revenue associated with it.

Emphasize that inventory management is a factor in providing high-quality veterinary medicine at an affordable price. Making this perspective a core element of the business is part of creating a "best practice" model for patients and clients.

Some practices get responsible staff members involved in assisting with inventory management by creating zones within the facility, with zone managers responsible for selected areas of the clinic. This creates a second level of inventory management, in which zone managers report to an inventory manager, and allows for better communication between the two about inventory expenses, expiration dates, and the need to manage their respective products to improve inventory management and cash flow for the practice.

Be sure to create ways to solve problems associated with inventory management. The sense of urgency and importance may be great, but developing lasting strategies to implement change is more important. The nature of the culture of your practice will aid in developing plans for improving communications and managing inventory better in the future.

17

How do I improve staff compliance, especially when staff members are busy?

Training is the cornerstone of a successful practice, especially in inventory management. First, educate the staff on the importance of inventory management. Show them the financial impact of product purchases versus product sales, and the impact on their compensation and benefits and on the growth of the practice. Hold frank, open discussions of how much products cost, how the practice structures its fees, and how charging clients properly for services and inventory items helps the practice.

An inventory manager is not merely the one ordering product and entering the data into the computer. He or she is responsible for training staff members on the proper way to enter inventory product sales on client invoices. You should have a written protocol, but continual training ensures that everyone is on the same page.

It is important that the job description for the inventory manager include training the staff on the proper way of doing tasks related to inventory. The manager needs to understand the inventory module software and be able to easily educate other staff members on all aspects of inventory management. One way to do this is to schedule periodic training sessions for each department in the hospital.

Make training a priority *and* a continual process. There will always be software enhancements that mean the staff will need more training. It also might be worth implementing a reward program to recognize and encourage compliance. Gift certificates to restaurants and shops are a great incentive with minimal cost to the practice.

18

How can I keep the inventory log up-to-date when people sometimes put things in the book without checking inventory stock first?

A well-managed inventory system will have protocols in place for tracking items in the practice. Establish a central stocking area—a central pharmacy—so inventory is not spread throughout the facility and everyone knows where to find additional products. If what is on the shelf is all the available stock for that product, it becomes obvious when the reorder point has been reached. If, on the other hand, you have product "X" on the pharmacy shelf and backup bottles in other locations in the clinic, failure or inability to check inventory stock will occur on a regular basis.

If you have assigned someone the role of inventory manager, that person can be responsible for double-checking the log and order book against stock before making an order, but improving the process will save time in such efforts in the future.

No matter how well your computerized or paper inventory control system functions, there is no substitute for routine physical counting of stock. You do not need to count stock every week or month, but you should become visually aware of what and how many items should be in your stocking areas. Often, if one person is doing the ordering, that person knows if the item on the want list is in stock, and where to look for it. The key is to develop this component of an inventory management program in your practice.

19

How do I educate new staff quickly?

There is no quick or easy way to teach someone inventory control, but having a formal system in place with written documentation is a major step in making it easier for a new person to learn what goes where and when to order new supplies. An employee manual is one way to establish and support training in this area.

All training should have standard operating procedures (SOPs) in writing. These become a quick reference guide for the new employee. It is advisable to schedule testing, both written and by demonstration, with training of all new hires. This improves compliance with how the practice does tasks. Quality training will lead to quality employees.

Training should never be limited to the first day of employment. Employees need to be continually reacquainted with different aspects of their jobs and retrained when new techniques become available or problems become noticeable. A mentoring program for all new hires is an excellent training option. This will translate book training into day-to-day, real-life situations. Mentorship starts with employees who enjoy teaching others how to accomplish their tasks. Those staff members can demonstrate the importance of performing inventory duties properly and how doing so benefits both the staff and the practice.

Because inventory training is a work in progress, give positive reinforcement for all efforts made toward understanding and using the system. The more any employee hears "good job," the more likely he or she is to continue performing up to expectations.

⇒ Do It Now

Write down three areas of inventory management you want all employees to know and understand. Then develop SOPs based on those three areas.

20

What is the most effective way to indicate reorder levels: tag system, computer reports, manual, or a combination?

There are at least three ways to develop reorder points: manual, computer-generated, or a combination of both. The comfort zone of the inventory manager leads to the most effective way to create and use reorder points, but a combination of physical and computer counts will generally create the best mix for determining reorder points.

If a practice does not have a software program, that limits its capabilities, as does having a computer that is weak on inventory control. There are numerous variations on the manual system. Most people rely heavily on the "red tag" system (see Question 1) to avoid the "oops, we ran out" problem. Another approach is to use an order board where staff members write the name of the product when they notice it is getting low. This information can then be double-checked against the tags to verify the product is, in fact, at its reorder point.

Other manual systems use a weekly physical audit of the inventory and order accordingly. This type of system (a zone system) uses a master sheet with reorder points, clearly indicated quantity on hand, and projected reorder levels, which will aid in creating the purchase order. Employing zone managers to count products and report their findings to the inventory manager will expedite the process.

The combination approach generally works best for most practices. They combine their software reorder reports with a quick visual assessment to confirm the accuracy of the report. For hospital-use inventory items, a weekly checklist indicates each item's reorder level. Some practices add a want list, often in conjunction with a tag system, as a backup to the computer system.

If the practice uses an inventory module for reorder, it is always wise to perform cycle counts to compare the accuracy of the computer with the actual products on the shelves. This will enhance accuracy by adjusting the computer inventory levels as a result of shrinkage.

⇒ Do It Now

Review your inventory management program to make sure you have checks and balances in place for maintaining reasonable accuracy of your inventory. Preventing shrinkage is a great first step in controlling inventory.

21

How do I get a large staff to understand the concept of reorder tags?

You must establish whether this is a training issue, the practice is understaffed, the present system makes little sense, or the staff is not being held to a high level of patient care, which includes maintaining the proper level of drugs and medical supplies. The solution to the problem starts with identifying the reason staff members' inaction.

If you find that training is the issue, reexamine your training program and make corrections as needed. Training begins with an understanding of the importance of having the needed product on hand to provide the quality of medicine the doctors are practicing. Point out all the reasons why the staff would be letting down the patient, the client, and the practice by not having the proper medications available for treatment.

You must train the inventory team properly. Make sure the inventory management have developed SOPs. Even if you have just a few, make sure they are available to all applicable team members. Then make time for team training and have the relevant staff members walk through the process of checking and reordering inventory with the whole inventory team.

Once you have completed the initial training, use the carrot-and-stick method for ongoing motivation: Make the staff feel that there is something in this for them. There can be a bonus—a "carrot"—if staff meet a certain goal related to inventory management. The bonus can be money, a gift certificate, or something else. The "stick" is writing someone up who did not follow the protocol, which can lead to dismissal.

This education or training is merely a step in making people accountable for their actions and reminding them that they are here to make the lives of pets and people better. Managers expecting change must be aware that it takes a minimum of two to three weeks to change employee habits. Staff need to be focused on their actions, and the inventory manager needs to be available for counseling during that time.

The problem may be the system—perhaps it needs to be replaced with something better. One option is to create a zone system whereby an individual is in charge of a zone. Dividing the practice into a few zones and creating zone managers makes it easier because you are dealing with a few individuals instead of the entire staff. A zone could be the treatment area, surgical area, diets, receptionist area, or controlled substances area. On a weekly basis, each zone manager performs brief physical counts of his or her products and reports the findings to the inventory manager, who in turn generates orders based on the supplies on hand. This system gives a more accurate accounting of the products on hand while streamlining the entire process.

Analyze the cause of the problem, and fix it. The practice cannot afford to let inventory get out of control. There are real reasons why the system is not functioning properly. The inventory manager should address the problem and be willing to make changes as needed.

22

How do we turn over ordering to staff members while helping them to resist those enticing giveaways from vendors?

Train staff to resist the temptation of freebies. If you have established an inventory manager, it will be easier to help staff do so because he or she will be who communicates with sales reps.

The owner or practice manager must establish organized training on the protocols for managing inventory, and dealing with freebies should be one of the elements of those protocols. This can mean free items go to the practice or inventory manager to handle, or even forbidding acceptance of freebies completely, in accordance with an SOP. Learning to say "no" is difficult, but can save the practice a lot of heartache and money.

Experience can be the best teacher in handling most of these issues. The manager needs to be mindful that not all deals, specials, or freebies are equal. Maybe giveaway items can be exchanged for better pricing on the product; such an approach comes from creating strong relationships with the sales forces of the companies involved. Another option is to create a budget for the inventory manager to follow. If the manager knows how much to spend and tracks how much has been spent, this can help turn freebies into better deals for the practice.

Whatever you choose, you need something in writing for staff to refer to when they are uncertain or under pressure from a salesperson.

23

How can we avoid wasting drugs and medical supplies?

To avoid waste, the team must help develop and implement an effective inventory management system. This will include discussions about rotating stock to ensure that dated products do not expire, are properly priced, and are monitored to reduce overstocking.

There also must be open communication among the inventory manager, doctors, and staff about the management system. This means having meaningful discussion with doctors about reducing the duplication of product lines for particular classes of drugs, and using a model in which a primary product and a secondary one are on hand instead of a full line of all products within a class of products. Such a system will aid in reducing overstocking. Consider creating an SOP for product additions. This allows for predetermined criteria to affect the decision about whether to bring more products into the inventory.

Educate staff to pay careful attention to details, such as filling prescriptions accurately and entering the proper quantities when dispensing products. This pattern of careful attention to detail must be applied to injection quantities and white goods, too. Consistent training of the technical staff will help create awareness of dosing accuracy and of the efficiency of inventory control measures.

One of the obvious ways to avoid wasting drugs and medical supplies is to create effective reorder points and reorder quantities that adequately factor in lead time (see Questions 7, 9, and 12). Since most products can be ordered to arrive at the office within a day, having a month's worth of a product on the shelves is counterproductive. Instead, maintain a quantity on hand that is adequate for about a two-week period. Next, use the inventory module in the practice management system, plus hand or visual counts, to ensure accuracy of current quantities. Order only when you have verified a product has truly reached its reorder point.

CHAPTER 3: DOCTOR BUY-IN

How do you get an owner-veterinarian to take inventory management seriously?

To convince the owner of the importance of managing and maintaining inventory supplies, good communication between the owner and inventory manager is crucial. The owner should request and receive regular updates on inventory budgets, supply levels, and unexpected expenditures, as well as shrinkage. This may sound easy and straightforward, but these update meetings must be scheduled and uninterrupted. If the owner is not on board regarding inventory, then managing the inventory will be a difficult challenge.

One suggestion for how to achieve this dialogue is to "show them the money." Inventory details are easy to gather and present as concrete proof of the need for serious management. Use the report module of the practice management software to generate usage, costs, and revenue for products; then use these reports to demonstrate where the money is going. Demonstrating the effect of managing inventory on the bottom line should gain an owner's attention. Remind the owner that inventory is money sitting on the shelf, and that it must be managed just like other cash assets. Be specific. Instead of saying, "We lost a carton of heartworm preventive," say, "We lost a carton of heartworm preventive valued at $490." Placing a monetary value on shrinkage should get an owner's attention, especially if you categorize it as lost profit.

Excellent inventory managers communicate the importance and value of inventory management to owners. Use as many resources as possible to demonstrate the amount of money sitting on the shelves and the vulnerability to shrinkage, if the inventory is not well managed. Be assertive and specific, and eventually you will get the owner to listen.

⇒ Do It Now

Start by setting up an initial meeting with the practice owner(s) or managers to discuss inventory management. Come prepared with what you would like to do with inventory, along with specifics about problems (including shrinkage), and get their feedback. Continue to set regularly scheduled meetings to discuss progress in inventory management.

What is the most effective way to get associate veterinarians to understand the concepts of effective inventory management and why we do not keep a specific product on the shelf?

Reports, open discussions with staff, and doctor meetings are all excellent ways to educate associate doctors about the importance of inventory control. The proof is in the numbers. Most recent graduates were not exposed to detailed training in inventory management while they were in school, so they need to be educated on its importance. Doctors tend to be analytical and visual; they need to see numbers, statistics, or some other visual proof to fully comprehend the importance of the information you are presenting.

Frank discussions regarding inventory management are essential. This is all part of mentoring young associates. For example, if a doctor insists on keeping a drug in stock that he or she dispenses only once or twice before it expires, calculate the true cost of the drug, the revenue generated from sales, and the waste from the expired product. Be sure to include shipping, taxes, and any other applicable costs associated with the product. This may convince a doctor why the item does not need to be stocked. Be sure also to suggest alternatives such as scripting a product out to a pharmacy.

Time should also be set aside at doctor meetings to discuss medications. If the consensus of the doctors is to add a new product, they need to decide what it will replace so the practice can "trade" one product for the other rather than retain duplicate inventory. The ground rule for any new product should be "If we add one, we drop one," and this needs to be spelled out at the beginning of every new employee's tenure, whether a veterinarian, an associate, technical staff, or a receptionist. Present this policy in an employee handbook and make it an element of inventory management protocols as well. This way, everyone knows the expectations.

Communication is the key to creating better awareness. Start with clear expectations from the beginning—make sure your doctors know about this aspect of your strategy for controlling inventory, along with other details.

How can we avoid having the veterinarians micromanage inventory?

To avoid having veterinarians micromanage inventory, make sure they trust the person who manages the inventory. Perhaps more importantly, have written protocols for inventory stocking, ordering, and receiving that they can review. Finally, use your veterinary management software to give the doctors monthly or quarterly inventory valuations, so they know how much money is truly sitting on the shelves.

Veterinarians need to be more involved in patient care and promoting the best-practice model than in inventory management. To accomplish this, schedule monthly doctor meetings to discuss medical records, protocols, and medications. The management team must set ground rules in advance for new or duplicate medications. The doctors must also realize that products are not an investment whose value will grow over time. Products are an asset for the practice that must be managed for optimum use and profit. Product selection is intended, by design, to improve the medicine the practice provides to patients based on patient need, not on "I want" demands. Make sure your doctors understand that product selection is evidence-based and items should never be stocked "just in case" they need them.

Accurate accounting of inventory should arrive at the value of inventory for your practice. Divide this number by the number of full-time-equivalent (FTE) doctors and you will have an average inventory for each doctor. The higher the number, the more cash the practice is tying up on the shelves. That is less cash to use for other activities.

Several organizations have published benchmarks for average inventory for a general practice per FTE veterinarian. The range is from $15,000 to $18,000 for drugs and medical supplies. Is this range ideal? Not necessarily. The more efficiently you can manage your inventory, the more you will be able to reduce the average inventory per doctor and free up cash for other activities in the practice.

A consensus must occur for the business side of the practice to meet the demands of providing quality, evidence-based medicine. The goal is healthy, happy pets and clients and a profitable practice. This means allowing doctors to do what they do best—medicine—while allowing the management team to do what they do best—manage the business. Micromanagement in any area, including inventory management, is unhealthy for the growth of the business.

27

How do you encourage veterinarians to make well-informed decisions about carrying new medications?

The first step in dealing with this challenge is to hold meetings to discuss cases. The next step is to reach a consensus regarding protocols for specific medical conditions whereby the use of certain drugs should be articulated. This is the point at which decisions should be made regarding which medications will be used; these decisions will become the foundation for limiting the number of drugs within categories of products. The discussions should include a defense of the proposed new medication: information about any research on its effectiveness and how many patients have been seen whose conditions suggest a need for the new drug.

The inventory manager and the management team need to establish policies related to how many products of the same category the practice will carry, and for how new products will be integrated into the inventory system. These guidelines and policies should be in writing and must be included in all discussions of medications by the doctors.

If the doctors elect to carry a new product, the guidelines for acquiring new products should be emphasized. As an example, for each new product, an older or underused medication will be eliminated from the inventory, either by using up present supplies or by returning the remainder of the unused product to the vendor for credit. Be sure to state in writing that allowing product to expire is wasteful and not acceptable.

Another solution when deciding whether to use a new medication is to "script it out" to an online pharmacy. Track the number of times this is done and how the patient responds. If doctors are using the scripted medication frequently and results are as good as predicted, then consider making it a part of the inventory.

➡ Do It Now

Develop a written policy for using new products. Include how a new medication will be purchased and evaluated for its effectiveness in treating patients. If it earns a place for future stocking, include a guideline on eliminating an existing product to make room in the inventory for this new one.

28

How do you get owners to let you know what they take home for themselves, family members, and neighbors?

If the policy of the practice is for all items dispensed or used by employees (owners are employees) to be recorded and invoiced, then everyone should follow the rules, including—perhaps especially—the owners, or they will undermine their leadership role. The inventory management system should include a form to show who has used what, when, and where.

Shrinkage is a major problem in all veterinary practices. It is not acceptable to have a double standard for shrinkage. If a staff member can be fired for stealing, an owner taking medication without invoicing or paying for it is also stealing and should be penalized. Having a different standard for an owner than for everyone else sends mixed signals to all, undermines morale, and actually encourages theft.

The practice should have a written policy about dispensing products for the pets of the practice owner and all staff. If the practice gives a discount or allowance to staff for treating their own pets, the policy should define the discount or type of allowance, and the allowance must be tracked via invoicing. Consider including how infractions will be handled. Once a policy is established and implemented, it sets the standard for the practice and makes it much easier to ensure that everyone is treated fairly.

A policy for dispensing medication to friends and neighbors should also be in place. First and foremost, a doctor/client relationship must exist before anything can be dispensed. This includes a medical record, with evidence of an examination of the pet or discussion by the doctor and the client regarding the patient, and which medication(s) are needed. With the legal relationship established, management must decide whether to give a discount for these special clients. The policy must be consistent whether it concerns a friend of the owner, of an associate doctor, or of a staff member.

These factors are important to ensure accuracy in inventory management. The precedent of proper invoicing of any product used in the practice or dispensed must be followed strictly and consistently. Without proper invoicing of quantities and accurate reorder points, it is impossible to manage inventory effectively.

How do I keep the associate doctors from giving away product or choosing not to charge for items?

The owner of the practice must establish a policy for this aspect of inventory and make it clear that the guidelines apply to all staff, including associate doctors. Educating all staff about the legal, financial, and tax consequences of faulty inventory management may not always have the desired impact, so occasional memos and training to reinforce this information are good ideas.

Remind associate doctors that any item dispensed through your practice's pharmacy or sold through your hospital must be recorded in the patient's medical history, and that this is a legal document in the event of a lawsuit. If a doctor chooses not to charge for a product, that is a discussion for you to have with that doctor, because it affects the profitability of the practice, the accuracy of your record keeping, and any potential legal conflicts (unapproved product giveaways could be considered as theft). The dispensed medicine must be recorded in the patient's medical records; however, if the decision is that the client need not pay for the item, have it discounted on the invoice.

Your practice is also liable for the sales tax on any product given away. Recording it on the patient invoice (which is part of the medical history) will deduct the product from your inventory counts, thus keeping inventory figures and sales tax liability records correct.

If the doctors are on a ProSal compensation, they need to be reminded that missed charges or discounts will affect their compensation. This should enhance their interest in tracking all their invoices.

If associates continue giving away product without practice approval, be sure to document this in their file because it is a serious offense.

In some cases, vendors may provide samples of certain products that can be used in lieu of the hospital's inventory. This creates some leeway in providing products at 100 percent discount. However, these samples must be recorded to ensure the accuracy of medical records and inventory.

Another approach is to offer doctors a monthly allowance or stipend for products or services they choose to give away, which can be spelled out in their employment contract. This lets them feel they are giving back to the community. These products will still be invoiced to keep the inventory counts correct, track the dollar value of such giveaways, and deduct from their stipends. The caveat is that any product or service doctors give away above the specified dollar figure will be deducted from their bonus. This will help them realize that everything affiliated with the practice comes with a cost.

⏵ Do It Now

Schedule a meeting with the owner or manager to discuss how to stop doctors from giving products away. Come to the meeting with possible solutions and ask for permission to develop a policy to address the problem.

How do you prove that employee theft is going on?

Before assuming that discrepancies in inventory are the result of employee theft, be sure to check the situation. Some discrepancies may be the result of carelessness or lack of a formal inventory management process. Theft is a serious accusation and should not be made lightly or without concrete proof.

If practice owners or managers are reluctant to respond to proof of theft, there may be little you can do other than accept the situation or move to another practice. It is the owner's practice, not yours, and the owner is ultimately responsible for its profit or loss.There are ways to present the gravity of the problem.

Try telling the owner about what is happening within the practice. Use inventory reports to show that profit is decreasing because of shrinkage. Doctors tend to want evidence-based information, and such information also is vital for any action taken against an employee over theft. Draw up the evidence as a spreadsheet with quantity ordered, cost per unit, retail price, and projected profit. Then do the same for actual usage with the actual profit. The difference is shrinkage, which may be attributed to theft. Use the evidence you have gathered to emphasize that theft may be an issue for the practice. Such cost accounting should get the owner's attention.

Tactfully remind the owner that loss of certain products, such as controlled substances, can have both a financial and a legal impact on the practice if there are discrepancies. The fear of a large penalty, especially related to the loss of controlled substances, can do a lot to convince owners that a problem exists and improved compliance is needed.

Merely being the messenger may not be enough to change anything, so bring solutions to the meeting. A formal action plan for reducing shrinkage and theft can go a long way in the process.

The next issue to address is follow-through. Will the owner give the inventory manager or practice manager the authority to make the changes on his or her behalf? Start with facts and end with a request for action. Most doctors are trained to collect facts to arrive at the best possible solution to a problem, so if you come prepared with the facts and a logical solution, you will likely gain their support. When you offer a way to potentially correct the problem, show on paper how this will reduce the shrinkage and enhance profits for the practice.

Be creative in your approach to educating the owner or manager and fixing the problem, but remind yourself that, if change does not occur, you still have the choice of staying or moving on to a practice that cares about this issue.

31
How do we identify worthwhile new products to bring into our practice?

Use a multilevel approach to determine new products or services to add to the practice. Let company representatives share information, but also use resources such as professional journals, veterinary-specific chat rooms, and other peer reviews to learn more about new products. Look at the economic impact a new product or service could have on the practice as well.

Information from drug representatives is an excellent resource, but cannot stand alone. Gathering enough information for a full picture may be the responsibility of one of the doctors or the practice manager. The more information that can be acquired, the more informed the decision will be.

If the potential new product is not a prescription drug, consider having the technical staff research and review the literature regarding the product and present their findings to the staff at a client service meeting. Ask them to include the pluses and minuses of the product, and ask for a tentative plan for marketing the item to clients and educating staff about the item if the practice elects to stock it. If the new product is similar to something presently on the shelves, be sure to include a discussion of how the old stock will be replaced by the new product.

Once a new product has been identified, ask the veterinarians to discuss its merits so they can reach agreement on its benefits for their patients and clients. Once a decision is made to try the product, buy small quantities and give the product a two- to three-month trial to determine whether it fits the needs of the practice and benefits patients. If the veterinarians review the results and agree that it is a product they would like to carry, they need to decide whether it will replace another product currently being stocked.

As new drugs or other inventory items are introduced, how do we house them in a limited-space pharmacy?

There is no need to stock multiple drug items that perform the same or similar functions. Everyone, especially the doctors, should agree to use only one or two drugs, at most, that do the same thing. If you stock something new, then by following the agreed-upon guidelines, something old must go.

Frequently checking usage reports will help you determine whether to keep an old item. Doctors have a tendency to think they use every product "all the time," but an effective inventory management system can provide evidence that an item is used only a limited number of times in a given year. Limited-use items do not warrant a place in your limited-space pharmacy. A solution would be to script this item out to your online pharmacy or to a local pharmacy, rather than to keep it on the shelf, taking up space with the potential to expire before it is used.

You may need to set lower reorder points, ordering smaller quantities more frequently, similar to "just-in-time" ordering (the ability to receive products when needed, as opposed to stockpiling product as inventory). Just-in-time ordering is an effective inventory efficiency tool, but may not be appropriate for all items on your shelves, especially with your most used items, where there is an increased risk of running out of stock. Using lower reorder points requires revisiting your inventory management protocol on monitoring and ordering products. If you need to modify your monitoring system, consider changing to zone counts (see Question 20). Reorder points and reorder quantities may not fit the formulas from Questions 7, 8, or 9, as your goal is to order less more frequently.

You may also need to reorganize the stockroom and the pharmacy. If you are not able to create a central pharmacy with only one entrance/exit to store products, then it is time to reorganize your shelves. Find a secure cabinet or closet, or an area that can be fenced in, to become your locked storage for at least your monthly heartworm and flea products.

Beyond separating your high-volume, high-dollar products from the rest of the inventory, organize your shelves in a logical manner and identify duplicate products. Ask the veterinarian to decide which is their primary product and script out for the other.

Finally, keep your inventory well organized. Reorganizing space can make it easier to manage inventory and/or create reclaimed space for a service or new piece of equipment.

CHAPTER 4: BENCHMARKS AND PRICING

33

How should I balance markup on the less expensive drugs versus the bigger-ticket items?

There are multiple factors to consider when determining markups on products. First, decide whether the product is a highly competitive one that clients might price-shop on the Internet or with other sources. Then consider whether the practice really needs to order and stock that item or whether it could be outsourced to an online pharmacy or obtained through a script written to a local pharmacy. Look at generic versus brand name as well. In cases where the generic is truly comparable to the brand-name version, the markup on the generic could be higher by instituting a minimum charge.

The majority of the respondents to the 2009 AAHA inventory management survey reported a base markup of 150 to 200 percent. From this starting point, they adjust markups in certain categories of products. For the highly competitive heartworm and flea/tick products, consider lowering the markup to less than 100 percent. This level of markup makes the practice highly competitive with other veterinary practices and with online pharmacies.

Some products you supply to clients via your online store may be priced competitively compared with retail outlets. This reduces the amount of product to be stocked and eliminates indirect costs, storage, and labor, while allowing for a fair markup. It also creates another profit center (similar to those for vaccination, surgery, etc.) for the practice.

The less expensive products, such as generic prednisone, may be marked up at a higher percentage. This can be accomplished by establishing a minimum-charge policy for the practice, which means the fee charged for a product will not be lower than the minimum charge. This automatically creates a higher markup on some products.

The goal for any practice is to achieve a balance between product and service sales. Most practices are becoming less reliant on product sales than in the past. The benchmark for the balance is closer to an 80:20 (service to product) ratio versus the 75:25 split of just a few years ago.

➡ Do It Now

Take the most recent year-end report from your practice management software and determine the percentage of gross revenue from product sales (excluding food) versus services. Ask yourself and your colleagues how you can improve on those numbers.

34

Are there different turnover ratios for different inventory items (e.g., antibiotics versus dewormers)?

Inventory turnovers for the entire stock should be a minimum of 10 to 12 times a year, but different products may turn over more or less frequently because of usage. The ratios for emergency items that are not used frequently will be lower than for packages of heartworm or flea/tick products. Ordering a 30-day supply makes the most sense from a financial perspective, because a practice can sell the inventory before it has to pay for it.

The strategy for increasing your turnover ratio is to know the usage of products (see Question 36). This is accomplished by reviewing the usage report from the practice management software. Then set the reorder points and reorder quantities based on usage, seasonality, and any other criteria you deem necessary (for reorder point formulas, refer to Questions 7 and 8). Remember that by adjusting usage, decreasing lead time, and decreasing order quantity, you will increase your turnover ratio. Once these steps are in place, monitor the results and make corrections when necessary.

A practice may find the same product is offered by a local pharmacy as a $4 script. If that is the case, you may choose to carry a smaller or starter size until the script can be filled at the local pharmacy. This reduces the sizes and quantities of products on hand, which can improve your overall turnover rate.

Some practices use pharmacy stores or online pharmacies on their websites to handle certain products. This still allows some financial return for the practice while eliminating the need to stock the product and keeping turnover at zero.

Improving product turns will improve the efficiency of the system and improve cash flow for the practice, but you still want to

BENCHMARKS AND PRICING

keep a product's usage and the practice's need of it in mind when looking at reorder points, order quantities, and turnover ratios.

How much inventory per doctor is adequate?

Most practices suggest having inventory levels on drugs and medical supplies of $15,000 to $18,000 per full-time-equivalent (FTE) doctor. These are suggested levels, but should not be considered as an ultimate level. The goal should be to determine the optimum level for your practice and to make adjustments as conditions change in the economy or at the practice.

An accurate physical count of inventory will help establish the ideal level for a given practice. Start by performing a physical count at least annually and then determining the total cost of the products. Divide that number by the number of FTE doctors to arrive at the inventory value per doctor. At the same time, compare actual product levels with corresponding quantities shown by the inventory management system and, when necessary, adjust your computer inventory quantities to match actual levels. This is yet another instance that underlines the importance of making regular, consistent entries in the inventory management system and on client invoices.

Another factor to consider is buying habits. If the practice can order as needed because of local warehousing and same-day delivery, the inventory per FTE doctor should be lower. If the practice is in a remote area, where delivery time may be a couple of days, the inventory level per doctor will be higher. Understanding your location and buying needs will help you determine an optimum inventory level for the practice, and consequently for the FTE doctors.

Yet another consideration is the type of practice. If the practice focuses strictly on wellness, with a limited number of sick patients, the level of products needed will be lower than for a busy critical-care type of facility, where the level of inventory will be higher because of greater demands for product.

The best approach to defining "adequate inventory" for your practice is to base the level on objective findings rather than on industry benchmarks or arbitrary suggestions.

▥➤ Do It Now

To find the average inventory per FTE doctor, do the following. Take your last full inventory count (cost of products on the shelves), or ask the practice manager for the number reported on the end-of-year balance sheet. Divide this dollar amount by the number of FTE doctors to arrive at the average inventory per FTE doctor. Remember, a FTE doctor works 40 hours per week. If you have two part-time doctors who each work 20 hours per week, together they may be considered as one FTE doctor.

How often should drugs turn over?

Every practice is likely to have a slightly different philosophy regarding the turnover of products. Factors affecting frequency of turnover include practical considerations such as the location, size, and type of practice, as well as philosophical considerations such as risk or comfort levels and experience of the inventory manager.

Although the inventory manager's experience has an immense impact on the number of turnovers, ultimately the owner or manager has the final say on which products to stock, and at what quantities. Progressive owners and managers realize that inventory control is important for the well-being of the practice, and will recommend more frequent turnover of products.

To determine the best frequency for turning over medications, start with the number of turnovers for the entire product line as of now (see Question 38). This gives you a baseline for measuring your success. Do the same thing for the "A" products (the high-use- or high-dollar-generating products). This provides two pieces of information with which to measure and fine-tune your product turnover. Set your goals for the number of turnovers for the year for "A" products, as well as for the entire inventory, and keep in mind that an inventory turn goal of 10 to 12 is reasonable for most practices.

Create a strategy for achieving these goals, then reassess your turns on a quarterly basis and make adjustments as needed to achieve your goal. Continue with this process until you believe you have optimized your time, space, and funds.

37

What dollar amount of inventory is ideal to have sitting on our shelves?

The dollar amount of inventory on the shelves is determined by several factors. The first is the type of practice and the number of doctors on staff. A vaccine clinic will have different needs than a 24/7 critical-care facility. Determine your practice type to start determining the dollar amount you need to keep on the shelves.

The second factor is your inventory system. A practice that has honed its inventory management so it is turning inventory 12 or more times a year will have less on the shelves than a practice that has elected to turn inventory 6 times a year. A practice that does not run out of products and runs close to "just in time" (see Question 32) will maintain a much lower inventory value on the shelves than one that does not have its inventory management under control.

The third factor to consider is the philosophy of the practice regarding inventory. If the practice owner or manager feels that writing scripts to online or local pharmacies is in the best interest of the patient and client, inventory levels will be very low. A practice that sees tracking orders, storing, controlling shrinkage, and return on asset as a nuisance may elect to have less controlled inventory. The practice that turns products frequently will have better cash flow than the practice that elects to have a year's supply of product on hand. The choice is the owner's.

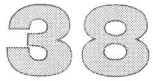

What is the best way to track turns in pharmaceutical inventory?

Every practice can easily track turnover, or turns, of all its pharmaceutical products or of a specific product. To do so involves use of "turnover ratio," which is a measure of the number of times a practice's inventory (either drugs and medical supplies or a specific product) is replaced during a given time period. The ratio is calculated as the cost of drugs and medical supplies (the actual cost a practice pays for the product or products) divided by the average cost of these inventory items during the same time period. The formula comprises two steps and is calculated as follows:

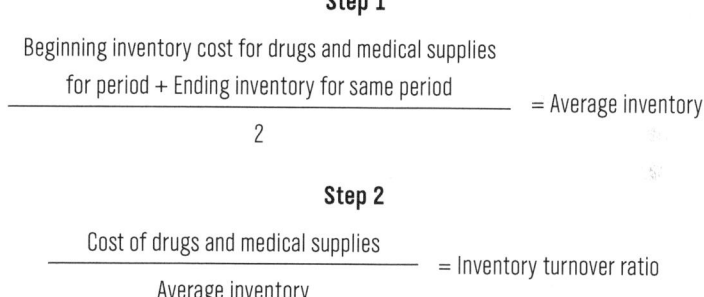

You can track turns of the entire inventory of drugs and medical supplies for the practice for a year. As an example, let us say you perform a full count of all drugs and medical supplies in the practice on January 1, and the actual cost of these items is $40,000. You perform a full count of all drugs and medical supplies again on December 31, and find you have $30,000 worth of items in the practice. To find the average cost of inventory for the year, add the beginning value ($40,000) with the ending value ($30,000) and divide by 2. The average inventory of these items is $35,000 ($40,000 + $30,000 ÷ 2 = $35,000). You have the average inventory and have completed Step 1.

BENCHMARKS AND PRICING

To complete Step 2, start by finding out how much the practice spent on drugs and medical supplies for the same time period (in this case, the year). You can request this financial data from either the practice manager or the bookkeeper. If the total amount spent on drugs and medical supplies for the year was $420,000, then divide it by $35,000, the average inventory you calculated in Step 1, to calculate the number of turns of the entire inventory of drugs and medical supplies. The equation would look like this:

$$\frac{\$420,000}{\$35,000} = 12$$

This means the entire inventory of drugs and medical supplies turned 12 times during the year. If your goal was to turn your entire inventory 12 times a year, or once a month, you accomplished your goal.

As mentioned, you can use this formula to calculate the turnover of a specific product, e.g., flea products. Following is an example of how to determine the turnover of a flea product for a year.

After performing a full count of flea products at the beginning of the year, you determine you have $5,000 worth of items (the actual cost of the product) in the practice. At the end of the year, you perform another count and have $3,000 (again, actual cost) of the same product. The average cost of the product for the year (the period of time) is $4,000 ($5,000 + $3,000 ÷ 2 = $4,000), which completes Step 1 of calculating turnover ratio.

Step 2 is to find the total cost of the product (actual dollars spent to buy the product) for the same time period as in Step 1. First total all vendor invoices for the product. If you determine the practice bought $48,000 of flea product during this period, you can apply the second calculation of the formula to arrive at 12 turns of the product ($48,000 ÷ $4,000 = 12).

Turns, or turnover, are easy to calculate for a specific product or for an entire inventory of pharmaceuticals. The more you can turn an inventory item or items, the less shrinkage (loss) will occur, and the less inventory there is to manage. Good turns also improve cash flow for the practice by tying up less money in inventory.

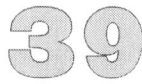

What percentage of revenue should the practice spend on drugs and medical supplies?

Each practice has its own culture and practice philosophy to help determine benchmarks to measure against. Start by making sure the practice is using a veterinary-specific chart of accounts (as published by AAHA Press) that separates expense categories such as diets, drugs and medical supplies.

To determine expense percentages for expense categories, divide dollars spent in a category by gross revenue. As an example, if your practice spent $200,000 on drugs and medical supplies and had a gross revenue of $1,000,000, the percentage of revenue spent in this category would be 20 percent ($200,000 ÷ $1,000,000 = 20%).

The benchmark quoted most often for drugs and medical supplies is 15 percent. Included in this category are drugs, white goods, needles and syringes, surgical supplies, and radiology supplies at approximately 10 percent and monthly heartworm/flea products at 5 percent. Diets and over-the-counter products are typically separate line items on the expense side of the income statement, and amount to 3 to 4 percent.

The goal is to budget drugs and medical supplies to 20 percent or less, eventually reaching the above-mentioned benchmark of 15 percent. To achieve these benchmarks will take patience and effort, and will require that you develop the protocol that best fits your practice.

Start by determining the dollars spent in this category last year and divide gross revenue for the same period by that amount to determine the percentage spent by the practice. If the percentages or dollar figures are not ideal, begin the process of creating a strategy for achieving better results. Create an action plan that incorporates specific goals, realistic outcomes, steps to perform, methods to monitor the steps, and time lines for the entire project.

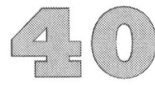

Does having a price on each item improve sales?

Whether having a price on each item improves sales may depend on the practice's philosophy. There is no hard evidence to prove or disprove this. You could survey your client base to find out which system they prefer and use those data as the basis of your decision.

On the pro side, if items in the point-of-sale area have prices listed on their packages, it allows clients to decide whether to purchase an item on this trip or the next one, depending on their current finances, without feeling obligated to get it now. It is when clients are at the practice that they are thinking about the immediate need for an item, so it makes sense to have the price available on the package. Such items are leashes, over-the-counter medications, and some of the monthly heartworm and flea/tick products.

At the same time, the practice needs to be careful when placing prices on products. The practice is obligated to have accurate prices, which means keeping track of product price changes. If a price has changed but the price on the package has not been updated, the price on the package should be honored. Charging a price different from what is on the package is a "bait and switch" offense that will result in client dissatisfaction and distrust; it is even illegal. Having a good inventory management system in place will ensure that prices on items are current and match what fees the computer shows as appropriate.

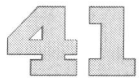

When and how much should we increase prices on inventory?

There are several factors to consider regarding inventory pricing and when to make adjustments, which usually means making a price increase. First, in general, consider the practice's pricing strategy. In your inventory, there will be shopped, value-added, and infrequently used items. Each category of items should have a different pricing strategy. The shopped items, such as monthly heartworm or flea/tick products, may be marked up 80 to 100 percent because of the highly competitive market for these products. The value-added products, such as antibiotics, may be marked up 125 to 175 percent. The infrequently used products may be priced much higher to ensure a return on investment equal to the projected value of the entire sale of a bottle of antibiotics, even if it may be used only once a year. Increases can be tied to what the practice is charged by its vendors, but you need those statistics to determine when and how much to raise prices.

Second, consider whether there has been shrinkage of a product and, if so, how much. Markups should include this factor to ensure the business receives the calculated return on its investment. If you believe that the markup levels suggested above cover your anticipated shrinkage, leave the levels as they are. If you wish to add to them, that is your choice. One reason for controlling and preventing shrinkage is that it can help your practice avoid raising prices on products, which clients will appreciate.

Vendor increases will occur on an annual basis at least and need to be monitored carefully. If you are using practice management software, the fields for each product should include a preset percentage markup. If you use this setting, the program will automatically mark up the cost of the product for you; each time you enter a new cost, a new price will be calculated automatically for the product. If you get special pricing and the price per unit goes down, you can override the calculated price for the older, higher price. The reason is straightforward: You negotiated the new cost, so you deserve the additional profit from the product.

On an annual basis, revisit your pricing strategy for all inventory items and determine whether the markup is adequate for the product. If you have found that shrinkage is different from that of the previous year, alter your markup percentage to reflect this change.

Markups typically stay the same for a year. It is the cost of the products that should be tracked and monitored. A good software program will do all the work for you as you or your colleagues enter new data.

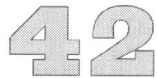

When figuring out markup on drugs and supplies, what should be included?

There is no right or wrong way to arrive at the true cost of a product or what markup to use, but the elements included in determining the price must mesh with the philosophy of the practice. All products have associated multiple costs to be considered. One of these is the cost of the product plus a prorated share of shipping expenses and applicable taxes. Some practices also include indirect costs in determining the cost of a product and how to mark it up, such as labor and storage expenses associated with merchandise.

Your inventory management program may or may not calculate shipping and taxes per item. If not, you may need to calculate the appropriate costs per product and include those expenses with the cost of the product. Once these numbers are entered, the program should calculate the selling price based on your already-established markup.

If you also choose to enter the indirect costs associated with products, you will need to add these values manually to the initial cost of the product, then enter them into the inventory management program. Another approach is to increase the markups by an additional percentage to cover these costs.

Everything done or used in a veterinary practice comes with a cost. All costs should be associated with some type of return. In the case of products, all costs should be accounted for, with a profit calculated in addition to those costs.

Veterinary medicine is a business and, as in so many other businesses, ancillary services come with costs. The end users—the clients—must feel they received their money's worth for the service or product.

Is it better to buy prepackaged or bulk and repackage, from a cost and liability perspective?

From a cost and liability perspective, many practices prefer to buy inventory items that are prepackaged. Using prepackaging allows staff to spend more of their time on patient care and client satisfaction. It addresses the liability issues in repackaging product, which is becoming an increasingly important issue.

Bulk is less costly initially, but think about the additional time staff need to separate and relabel bulk items and whether they are doing it properly. Total cost will be similar to that of buying prepackaged items. Many practice owners and managers feel that having all the information sheets present with each prepackaged product is a safety net, in terms of both legal liability and client education, that is worth the initial cost difference.

The number of lawsuits over the process of repackaging of bulk items is on the rise. Make sure you have reviewed the regulations on this topic, at both the state and federal levels, before buying bulk products for repackaging. Problems in this area can result in fines and bad publicity, which could ruin a practice.

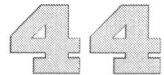

Is it more cost-effective to use online pharmacies to fill some product orders than to carry in-house inventory for all dispensing needs?

First, let us distinguish between online and Internet pharmacies. Online pharmacies are those to which the practice subscribes to handle some product sales, whereas Internet pharmacies market directly to clients and are privately owned.

There are two schools of thought on whether using online pharmacies to fill some product orders is more cost-effective than carrying in-house inventory for all dispensing needs. One is that it makes sense to use online pharmacies for some products, while the other is that doing so means losing control of the profit and/or client.

Online pharmacies are a double-edged sword. They are convenient for clients, but the veterinary practice misses out on the entire sale. For noncritical or specific drugs that are slow sellers, items that are used only occasionally, and/or drugs that often expire before the bottle is used up, online pharmacies are a great option. If you have a large client base, it does not make sense to carry one product for just one client. Consider adding an online pharmacy to your inventory management system for expensive, hard-to-obtain products, or for special-order items.

Some argue that it takes more time to use online pharmacies, which can lead to less profit for the practice. That can be true, but the counterargument is that the practice is still making money without the headache of data entry and the need for space to stock the product. Handling fewer products can allow the practice to use the freed-up space for new equipment or a new or expanded service. Profit from a service is usually higher than from a product sale.

You could also argue that stocking all products keeps the door swinging with more clients visiting the practice, which can generate additional services or product sales. This may be true, but sometimes the cost of handling slow-moving products may not be worthwhile. An alternative is to be helpful and educate clients about how your online pharmacy will benefit them. Ultimately, a client who is well informed about products and services may seek additional service because of a stronger bond with the practice.

The ultimate answer to whether it is appropriate to use online pharmacies lies within the culture and mission of the practice. What do the doctors and staff believe is in the best interest of the patient, client, and practice? Review the practice's mission statement and then look at whether the use of online pharmacies fits the culture of the practice. If it does, be selective about the products you script out. If it does not, focus on managing your inventory carefully to ensure you are not losing valuable resources—money, personnel, and time.

➡ Do It Now

Find your mission statement and review it to see whether online pharmacies fit your culture. If you do not have a mission statement, there is no better time than the present to get the team started on creating one for your practice.

CHAPTER 5: ONLINE PHARMACIES

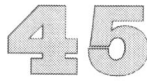

Have big pharmacies that offer common prescriptions at $4 affected which medications most veterinary practices stock and, if so, how?

Clients are cost conscious, especially in an economic downturn, and will ask if a script for medication can be issued. Progressive practices are embracing the concept of $4 scripts because it provides cost savings to clients and lessens the amount of product the practice purchases. Determine what will work for your practice by researching and developing strategies to adapt to the availability of products sold at $4. Doing so can be a win-win for your clients and for your practice.

The list of products on the $4 list is growing because people want to pay less for products. Most people do not realize that this is a tactic used by the retailer to bring in customers so they will purchase other items at regular prices.

Learn and understand the buying habits of your clients. Use the report module of your practice management software to create reports to determine dollars generated versus product usage over the past few years. Ask yourself if buying habits are changing and, if so, how. Practices that have felt the pinch have discontinued keeping some rarely used drugs in stock while writing more scripts to pharmacies. Knowledge of your clients' buying habits can help you identify whether this is an issue and, more importantly, how to handle it in the future.

Matching prices with retailers can be counterproductive for most veterinary practices. Instead of getting upset over the competition, create strategies that will benefit the patient, client, and practice. Consider creating an online "store" on your website that will compete with the lower prices from retailers and enhancing value by educating clients about the importance of using products approved

ONLINE PHARMACIES

for animals. Whenever possible, use the $4 script option from your local pharmacy.

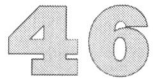

How does a practice justify fighting the Internet when inventory management is so costly and markup is so low?

Working against the trend of clients using the Internet to order products can be self-defeating. Veterinary practices are often small-scale operations challenging the large Goliath-type corporations that operate on the Internet. Internet pharmacies deal in volume to derive a profit margin. They have streamlined systems in place that allow for efficiency. They can buy in volume and negotiate price savings on products from suppliers.

Most clients want a medication at the time of service, so veterinary practice owners and managers need to find a balance between a sufficient markup to keep the business profitable and being aware of what online pet pharmacies charge. Ultimately, you cannot compete with Internet pharmacies, so make your services and professionalism, not your pricing structure, the reasons clients use your practice.

Keep in mind, by the way, that inventory management is only expensive when it is not used. Effective inventory management is an investment in the practice and, when done correctly, will save the practice money and increase its profitability, rather than add to its costs.

Rather than worrying about competing with Internet pharmacies, see whether you can apply aspects of the Internet pharmacy model to your practice. Streamline your inventory management system to include efficiency and cost savings to the client and negotiate pricing with vendors to improve your profit margins, when possible.

Medication sales are a highly competitive business and no longer an exclusive area for veterinarians. These sales should not be more than 23 percent of your gross revenue. The percentage has decreased over the past decade, partially because of Internet pharmacies, but more importantly because of the need to provide more hands-on services and outstanding client service. Veterinary practices are becoming less reliant on product sales while their net profits are improving.

Focus on providing services, education, caring, convenience, a personal touch, and professionalism that the Internet pharmacies cannot give customers. Your mission in practice should be to provide the highest-quality service and medicine for pets. Clients choose their veterinarians based on many factors. Some will seek the least expensive alternative for everything. Pet owners who use the Internet for medications often come to your office for veterinary services, so impress them with your care and professionalism. Remember, services have a higher profit margin than drugs.

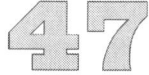

What are some ideas for starting up an in-clinic online pharmacy?

To launch an in-clinic online pharmacy, start investigating the online pharmacies available to your practice. Some are based on pet portal, while others can be added to your website, but will not allow the client to look at portions of a pet's file. Ask host companies for demonstrations and lists of current users, and check with users about how they like the system. Ask questions about available products, procedures for tracking and reporting usage to the practice, and how they would partner with your practice. Look for a provider that has an exceptional reputation with its veterinary users.

The entire experience for the practice and the client needs to be simple, seamless, and user-friendly. In providing this type of service to your clients, you want everything about the site and how the company treats clients to be in line with how you treat your clients—with compassion and care. The pharmacy becomes an extension of your practice, and clients will judge the practice, in part, on their experience with the pharmacy.

On occasion, the pharmacy may do a better job of handling a client's requests than your practice. Survey your clients to see how they like the website and the service it provides, and adjust the relationship accordingly. If the site is efficient and responsive and clients have reached it through your veterinary practice, it will reflect well on your practice and help you retain clients.

When setting up your online pharmacy, start by creating a list of products it will provide to clients and those it will provide only on occasion, not products that are imperative for starting treatment immediately. You may want to use the pharmacy for clients to order diets, which will reduce the need to order and store large quantities of food.

ONLINE PHARMACIES

Some practices use perks to entice clients to use their online pharmacies, such as a discount on a service or points toward a product of their choice. Promote the website wherever you can. This will draw more clients to the site for client education, upcoming events, and other promotions.

Management will need to draft a strategy for the type of usage desired from the website. It may be possible to reduce inventory to the bare minimum and use the online pharmacy for almost everything. Take the time to make an informed decision about the extent to which you want your online pharmacy to serve your clients and support or replace your inventory.

⇒ Do It Now

Go to the Internet and research several veterinary-specific online pharmacy companies to see what they offer. Ask them for references. Contact several of these and ask how they like the service. The more knowledge you can gain, the more informed will be your decision.

48

Should a clinic stock more than one category of drugs (e.g., nonsteroidal anti-inflammatory drugs)? If so, how many, and would using something like an online pharmacy be a better solution?

In determining whether to stock more than one category of drugs, such as nonsteroidal anti-inflammatory drugs (NSAIDs), the first decision depends on what the practice truly believes in. If the philosophy of the practice is to be all things to all people, then having an overabundance of products probably works. If, on the other hand, the practice believes in the best-practice model, then having a primary and a secondary product from the same category is the best choice.

In the latter case, doctors must decide which product is their primary choice, with a limited quantity of a secondary product to be kept in stock. An online pharmacy can offer a tertiary source of products.

By limiting the number of similar products to two, practices conserve the cost of inventory on their shelves, which helps in managing both cash and inventory. With the increasing number of alternatives for providing clients with products, there are fewer reasons to stock as much inventory as in the past. Online pharmacies can be an extension of your practice and save you the headache of managing more inventory. In most cases, using an online pharmacy means the practice can receive a profit on the sale of the product without the costs associated with ordering, storage, and shrinkage of additional products.

Thanks to $4 scripts and online pharmacies, both the client and the practice have more options for treating pets. The convenience factor to both is important, but not the only factor to consider. In some cases, cost can play the primary role in this process. If clients

ONLINE PHARMACIES

find a product offered at a lower price through an alternate source and it is approved by the Food and Drug Administration, let clients make the choice between your in-house pharmacy and another source. Do not worry about losing revenue from the lost sale of a product, because clients will always need your skills and knowledge of medical and surgical issues. Charge appropriately for your services and concentrate on providing the best service possible. Try to look at monies generated from the pharmacies (in-house and online) as extra profit for the practice.

ONLINE PHARMACIES

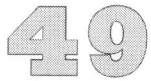

What are some creative ways of competing with Internet pharmacies?

There may be creative ways to compete with Internet pharmacies, but a practice is usually better off not trying to do so. Internet pharmacies have better buying power and require lower profits because of their volume sales. A practice may actually need to embrace the concept, perhaps by setting up its own online pharmacy on its website, of accommodating clients who always seek the least expensive approach for a product or service.

Instead of panicking or attacking, be supportive with clients interested in making purchases from Internet pharmacies. Recommend that they double-check products when they receive them for expiration dates, packaging issues, and correct dosages. Warn them, tactfully, that products from some Internet pharmacies may not have been manufactured to the standards required by domestic government agencies. Give them the pros and cons so they can make a choice. They will always remember that you helped them by providing excellent service.

Lowering prices simply to compete can be dangerous, but sometimes it can be beneficial to the practice. With the advent of $3 and $4 prescriptions for certain generic drugs, you may elect to price these products similarly. Take a service such as a wellness program and offer a lower price for a monthly product if the client elects to purchase the entire program. This lowers the price of the product to gain compliance with the program. Remember that services generate more profit than products do. In this case, the entire value of the wellness program is far greater than a little lost profit on a product sale.

For some of your in-house programs, your vendor may supply free product in exchange for ordering more of the product. The challenge is to be creative in how you use the free goods while tying them to services.

ONLINE PHARMACIES

50

Should we stock nonprescription products that can be purchased through an online pharmacy?

It is reasonable to consider stocking nonprescription (nonscript, for short) products in limited quantities that can be purchased through online pharmacies. Some clients prefer to purchase products directly from you for the convenience, out of trust, or because they lack access to a computer. The practice needs to serve such clients, but should be cautious about overstocking because the goal is to manage and balance three key assets: product, labor, and money.

Do limit the quantity of over-the-counter items kept in stock. It is worthwhile to stock items such as ear cleanser and cat laxative that would be dispensed during a medical-problem visit. If a product can be purchased easily from a local pet store, though, consider not offering it and referring the client to the appropriate store. For the most part, limiting the inventory of products the client can acquire from other sources is a good idea.

Survey the practice inventory and determine which nonscript products have multiple sources for clients. Then decide which ones to carry and which ones the client should purchase from an alternative source. Knowing which products have multiple sources, researching the options for the client, and making an informed decision on whether to handle the product makes it easier to manage inventory efficiently and potentially frees up cash for other needs.

With such information in place, the practice can tell the client, "Yes, we have it, but the cost may be higher than at the pet store." If you can provide an alternative, the practice still has a chance for the sale. For some clients the convenience of getting it now outweighs driving to another location and spending more time to save a few cents, or even spending the time to go online to obtain the product. It is ultimately the client's choice.

51

What quantities of an item sold warrant keeping the item in inventory?

Frequency of sales and quantity sold are excellent starting points in determining whether it is worth keeping an item in inventory. The inventory manager should evaluate each item in inventory on a case-by-case basis annually to determine whether sales warrant stocking it. Develop and implement a protocol that defines the parameters for product selection, which may include how critical the product is for the practice, a projected price for the product, and projected frequency of turns. If a product is critical for the practice and turns once a year, it may be worthwhile to continue stocking it. If, on the other hand, the product is not critical for patient care and turns infrequently, consider making it a special-order item or writing a script to a pharmacy.

Any product on the shelves must be entered into the inventory management program, and its usage tracked. A usage report will identify products that turn only infrequently. Then research why the product has a low number of turns—slow turns may be due to setting too high a reorder point or infrequent use.

Quantity sold does not necessarily dictate whether you stock a product; sometimes it is the use for the product. A slow-moving product may be needed to treat a critical, life-or-death case.

Once you identify reasons for the poor performance, make adjustments as needed (i.e., to the reorder point). Use the inventory system for tracking and fine tuning what the practice needs and uses. Any item purchased, used, or dispensed warrants tracking in the inventory programs and determining whether to continue stocking it or find alternative sources for it.

ONLINE PHARMACIES

52

How can we keep our inventory cost down but still offer our clients cost-effective options?

Three factors are involved in keeping inventory down while delivering cost-effective options to clients. The first factor is having an inventory management plan that lets you optimize purchasing, selling, and profit from products. It is critical to implement a plan that allows for negotiating good prices from vendors while setting realistic reorder points and reorder quantities to conserve the indirect costs, labor, and storage. Doing this may mean your markups can be lower, making products more affordable for clients.

The second factor is reducing the duplication of products. This starts with a discussion among the doctors in order to arrive at a consensus on their need for a primary product for a given treatment plan and a small quantity of a secondary product, if necessary. Reducing duplication will improve cash flow and inventory management.

When possible, use alternate sources for some products. Use online pharmacies or local pharmacies for products used only once a year. Those prices may be lower than your in-house pharmacy prices, which helps the client. Be sure to let clients know when these options save them money.

The third factor is your pricing model for services and products. Services always generate more profit than product sales. By pricing services appropriately, a practice may be able to lower its markup on medications. This demonstrates the value of the skill and knowledge the veterinarians provide, while offering competitively priced products.

Start by evaluating your inventory management and pricing strategies. Look at the value perceived by the client and the actual profit associated with services and products. Then make pricing decisions based on benefit to the patient, the client, and the practice.

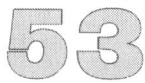

Will practices be more or less reliant on writing prescriptions to local and online pharmacies in the future?

The likelihood is that practices will become less reliant on stocking and dispensing products. For the past decade, the revenue generated from dispensed products has dropped by nearly 10 percent, partly because of the better pricing of services and partly because of reduced reliance on product sales for practice growth.

For a growing number of practices, the expense of drugs and medical supplies is at nearly 20 percent or less. Practices are managing inventory better than in the past and are evaluating programs that can help both the patient/client and the practice. Some of these sources are the $3 or $4 scripts at local pharmacies and online pharmacies.

The reality is that online pharmacies are growing in popularity. Linking them to the practice website means the practice still has some control over the products offered by the pharmacy. Online pharmacies let the practice script out for products they no longer wish to stock while retaining a portion of the sale price. By controlling the products prescribed and, to a degree, the purchase price, veterinary practices are embracing the concept.

Although this trend will not eliminate the need to stock certain products, practices are likely to become more reliant on outsourcing for most products. To cope with this situation, veterinary practices must focus on the services they provide as the core business elements offered to clients. Products are important and can bring in additional revenue and profit, but the margins on products are decreasing and, at some point, the cost/benefit will tilt more to other sources for dispensing products to clients. These sources are likely to be online pharmacies and your local drugstore.

CHAPTER 6: RETAIL CENTERS AND IN-HOSPITAL USE

What percentage of annual growth should a practice see in food sales?

First decide if your practice will handle and sell food products, or if it will outsource the majority of sales to its online pharmacy. If you elect to handle food, food sales are an important aspect of inventory and should generate a percentage of growth for the practice every year. A realistic annual percentage for growth in food sales, including both prescription and maintenance products may be as much as 5 percent. Or, if you consistently achieve the benchmark of 3.5 percent of gross food sales, your increase may be closer to the annual growth of the practice's gross revenues.

Your practice's percentage of growth from food sales may depend on the diets you carry. If you carry prescription-only diets, then growth expectations depend on your medical caseload and may be low. If your protocol for a medical condition includes a prescription diet, then your growth expectations may be high because food sales are linked to a medical protocol. If your food sales include maintenance foods, you may see more of a growth increase partly because of the wellness programs recommended by the practice, which may prescribe a certain type of food.

In assessing your practice's growth in food sales, one of the first factors to consider is the veterinarians: If the medical staff does not believe that specialty foods are important, growth of these products will be minimal at best. If the doctors believe in proper nutrition from puppy- or kittenhood to the geriatric stage and incorporate diets into wellness protocols, sales may exceed an annual growth rate of 5 percent.

Another factor to consider is whether you have a system in place to order, receive, and sell foods without tying up a significant amount of cash or storage space. The inventory manager must monitor quantities

RETAIL CENTERS AND IN-HOSPITAL USE

to make sure reorder points and reorder quantities are realistic and—better yet—that foods turn frequently. Turnover of food should occur at least 24 times a year or the profit margin will drop rather than increase. Frequent turns also mean fresher food.

To increase turns, some practices stock small starter bags of foods to dispense during visits and order larger maintenance sizes for clients to purchase. A designated staff member calculates the probable number of days a bag of food or flat of cans will last for clients, and based on that calculation, enters a reminder date into the inventory management system. About one week before the food should run out, a staff member calls or emails clients to ask how much food is left and whether the client wants to order more.

Once such a system is in place, the practice should be able to order and sell food before the vendor invoice must be paid. This increases the number of turns of food, bringing the system closer to "just-in-time" inventory management.

➡ Do It Now

Use your practice management software to total the dollar sales of foods purchased and foods sold for the past three years. Determine the percentage of change in food sales during this period. Use that information to decide the level of increase you want for the next 12 months and create a strategy to achieve that goal.

RETAIL CENTERS AND IN-HOSPITAL USE

What is the best way to prevent inaccurate sales of similar items (e.g., can versus case, one flavor versus another)?

Inaccurate sales of similar items is an issue for many veterinary practices. Preventing this problem begins with checking that all products have been entered in the practice management software correctly. The next step is to perform medical record audits by comparing the medical record with the client invoice. Audits help catch inaccurate entries, sales of similar items, and even missed charges. These efforts can also help identify problems with the inventory system or with certain staff members who need additional training. The inventory manager should keep an eye on the entire process and address problems quickly and assertively.

Training new hires and reacquainting the more experienced staff on how to enter information in the computer, whether for invoicing, medical records, or overall inventory management are of paramount importance. Make sure they become proficient in identifying the products and quantities dispensed. Continue training at regular intervals to reacquaint everyone with updates, new products, and new information.

The inventory manager will need to create a protocol for coding items for the computer. If available, you could use a barcode reader that reads the Uniform Packaging Code (UPC) on the package. Some inventory management programs have integrated barcode-reading software into their programs, and barcode scanning will be more common in the future.

The inventory manager also could develop a code system for foods. For instance, an item in a bag uses a code beginning with "B"; an item in a case uses a code beginning with "C"; and an item in a can uses a code starting with "K." The letters are followed by

RETAIL CENTERS AND IN-HOSPITAL USE

numbers or other letters. Be creative and consider getting the staff involved by asking for their input on a simple and effective way to distinguish among cans, bags, and cases.

The inventory manager also must be extremely familiar with the various fields for each product entry in the practice management software. The program may allow you to set up prices based on quantities dispensed. For example, the price for a can needs to be greater than merely arriving at a per can price by dividing the number of cans in a case by the case price. The reasons are the extra labor involved in opening a case; once a case is open and on the shelf, you can sell only individual cans and must do so before the food expires. Use the inventory program to identify the easiest method of accomplishing your pricing strategy, single versus a case price.

How do you determine a dispensing fee for pharmaceuticals?

Setting dispensing fees (a fee for preparing and dispensing certain drugs to clients) for pharmaceuticals is a constant challenge for a veterinary practice. It is not unusual to come up with a number at random and call it the dispensing fee. That number may derive from articles in veterinary publications that list benchmarks for dispensing fees, or merely from copying what a colleague charges.

Random pricing can be dangerous if you are not comparing similar practices, but you can derive an appropriate fee by using a simple equation that accounts for the practice's expenses and creates an appropriate fee.

To establish a dispensing fee, determine the average hourly rate for the technicians. Next ask the owner, manager, bookkeeper, or CPA for the percentage of gross revenues for nonprofessional staff members, which should be close to the benchmark of 20 percent. Finally, find out how long it takes for the practice to fill a script.

Let us say that the average technician hourly rate is $12, nonprofessional staff costs are 20 percent, and average time to fill a script is four minutes. At first glance, the time factor looks like four minutes, but it is actually eight minutes, because an equal amount of soft (training) time is needed for every minute of actual labor.

Eight minutes is 0.13 hour (8 ÷ 60 = 0.13). If you multiple 0.13 times $12, you have $1.56 in labor costs. Dividing $1.56 by 20 percent (nonprofessional staff costs) creates a dispensing fee of $7.80.

Setting a dispensing fee is easier than spending time finding out what colleagues charge, which could be considered price-fixing. The smart inventory manager figures out a dispensing fee specific to his or her practice.

RETAIL CENTERS AND IN-HOSPITAL USE

⏵ Do It Now

Conduct a time study to determine how long it takes to fill a prescription. Once you have the average time it takes to fill a script, find the average hourly wage for a technician. Use those numbers to calculate your dispensing fee.

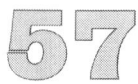

What is the most effective way to manage prescription diets, which take up a lot of time and space for a relatively low markup?

To manage this area, the veterinarians must reach a consensus about which diets they would like to prescribe, and the inventory manager should then research the most economical way of handling these items. Then formulate a plan that is cost-effective for both the client and the practice. Because of the low markup on foods, using and/or prescribing only one brand of kidney, intestinal, or other specialty diet is essential.

One method is to handle only the small bags of foods that are initially dispensed to clients, and then to order a bigger bag to arrive on a scheduled delivery day. The trick is to have a system in place that can meet future client needs quickly and efficiently. A computer recall system and approximations of how long a bag should last are helpful in developing an effective system. Calling clients to order what they need when they need it will cut down on the amount of diets (inventory) the practice must keep on hand.

Usage reports are helpful in that you can review the prior two years to see if there are trends in how much of a certain food was used. The analysis that comes from monitoring usage reports will help you order, and maintain, a two-week supply of a food type and adjust from there. This will keep the food fresh and payment coming in from clients before vendor bills are due.

There is an increasing interest in the use of online stores to handle food. The practice gives the client a code to order from its online store and the food is drop-shipped to the client. This has two advantages: The practice receives money from each sale and reduces its need to stock foods. The savings in improved cash flow and better use of space are definitely worth considering.

58

What is the easiest way to track in-hospital use of retail items (e.g., food)?

There is no easy way to track in-hospital use of retail items, including food. A lot depends on how the practice tracks inventory. Remember, all products used in patient care need to be accounted for, whether on the client's invoice or in some form of hospital account.

If possible, create a central pharmacy where access to products is only through a written requisition. This system is simple, straightforward, and much easier to track because there is either an invoice for a client or a requisition sheet for hospital use.

If your practice management software lets you set up a hospital account, do so. As the staff uses products, those products must be invoiced to the hospital account. The invoices are zeroed out when the quantity is invoiced from the computer. The hospital appears on the invoice as the provider. For verification purposes, make sure everyone is trained to initial the invoice upon removing the stock. If this method seems complicated, check with your software vendor and see if they can suggest a better way to approach this issue.

Another approach is to put clipboards on the shelves with inventory-use sheets that ask for the name of the item, unit size, number of items taken, and initials of the staff member taking the item. On a regular basis, use the sheets to adjust the record of quantities on hand in the inventory management program.

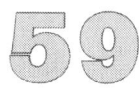

Should we include items like allergy tests and oxygen in our inventory? If so, where are those items tracked?

Some practices track items such as allergy tests and oxygen as inventory, while others place them in different categories—oxygen under "leased items," allergy testing kits under "lab," and so on. The choice of method for tracking these items is up to the inventory manager, practice owner, or manager. What is important is that the items are tracked formally in the first place.

As an example, if oxygen tanks are treated as leased equipment, the practice needs to know how many are on hand and when to order replacement tanks. The inventory or zone manager can perform a weekly audit of the tanks and order replacements when the reorder point is reached. For this inventory item, a visual audit is easier than tracking usage in the inventory module.

Set up allergy testing so a prepaid test is automatically removed from inventory when the client is invoiced for it. If the practice considers allergy testing items or heartworm tests as laboratory expenses and tracks them by visual counting, there is risk of miscounting and running out of items. Creating a category for these items in the inventory management software will head off this problem, and doing so also will track usage and link items to the service (e.g., allergy testing).

60

What are some tips for keeping our monthly flea/tick inventory straight in light of free-dose promotions?

There are two issues to consider when looking at keeping monthly flea/tick inventory up-to-date in light of free-dose promotions. The first is tracking free doses in inventory, and the second is ensuring that coupons accurately reflect the quantity of free product dispensed.

Start by training staff to enter these monthly products by tube in the inventory system; when you sell a three-pack, put "3" in the program. When the free-dose promotion is scheduled, enter it into your system as if it were sold to a client. Once it is invoiced, remove it from your inventory, but override the price and place a zero cost on the invoice. By entering all the dispensed items with the free ones listed as a zero charge, clients can see that they were given credit for the free-dose promotion. Some practice management software systems have addressed this issue by creating a "quantity" pricing setup. As an example, if the promotion is one free dose with every six, the pricing setup for seven doses will be the same as for six. Just remember to revisit the pricing module to readjust the setup after the promotion ends. Check with your software vendor to see whether this setup is available. If not, ask your vendor for the best way to perform this task.

Run a report at the end of each month for monthly flea/tick products sold and use that report to fill out rebate coupons. It saves time to do this all at once, and cuts down on missing rebate forms, which can occur if forms are filled out at time of purchase.

For the sake of inventory control, make sure the practice does a cycle count of selected products (e.g., heartworm and flea/tick products) at least once a month. The volume of sales for these products lends itself to a higher probability of shrinkage. Accurate counts of these products will help control their use and improve profitability. Make corrections when necessary to ensure that you know where all the product ends up, and you will have optimized your profit.

CHAPTER 7: INVENTORY CONTROL

61

How many times per year should we take physical inventory to make it easier at year-end?

Performing physical counts throughout the year makes record keeping easier at the end of the year; how often your practice does this depends on the number of people available to handle the task. The recommended minimum is twice a year for all products. An increasing number of practices perform quarterly cycle counts.

One way to perform the cycle counts is to divide the inventory into three areas. On a monthly basis, count one of the three areas, which means all areas are counted once per quarter. If you repeat the cycle each quarter, the entire inventory has a physical count four times during the year.

Some practices perform a quarterly physical count on the entire inventory but count retail and fast-moving products, such as heartworm or flea products, on a monthly basis. This approach provides better management of inventory of the fast-moving products and helps reduce shrinkage from theft or missed charges. Fast-moving items typically constitute a significant amount of the gross revenue from product sales, so it makes sense to count these products often.

Another approach is to establish zones and have a designated zone manager perform weekly counts of each zone. This tracks all products and allows for adjustments of items to be updated in your practice management software program; aids in identifying possible shrinkage issues, by comparing actual counts with computer counts; and gives you the current cost of inventory.

INVENTORY CONTROL

How can we control inventory costs from month to month?

Controlling inventory costs from month to month is a challenge, but an inventory management system will make it easier, even in those months that seem to be out of control. The first step is to consolidate orders to fewer vendors and work with these vendors to obtain excellent pricing contracts. Vendors are usually willing to work with you on pricing for guaranteed business. The next step is to pinpoint weekly usage of products in the practice. Once you get a handle on weekly usage of items, you can start to plan ahead.

Setting appropriate reorder quantities and reorder points is another way to control inventory costs. You should never have more than a four-week supply of any product. Reorder quantities and reorder points can be changed because of the seasonality of products. Good reorder quantities and reorder points typically allow the practice to sell the product before the bill is due.

You can also run usage reports from your practice management software. This will show you what was used and in what quantities during a specific period of time. Usage reports aid in determining reorder points and when to make seasonality corrections. See Question 7 for an example of a reorder point being adjusted for seasonality.

Some practices budget dollar amounts to be spent in any given month by employing benchmark percentages—16 to 20 percent of gross revenue—for drugs and medical supplies. The next step is to create a budget with monthly projections for revenue and to use these percentages to determine how much the practice could spend on a monthly basis for drugs and medical supplies.

Controlling inventory costs from month to month is a challenge. There are always unexpected situations (e.g., a run of parvo dogs or an unexpected shortage of a product), and trying to control inventory on a monthly basis can be a bust. When this happens, go back and see what you can adjust (i.e., reorder points, reorder quantities) to get back on track so quarterly costs are at what you projected. Inventory management is not an exact science: It is setting up methods that work most of the time and making adjustments when needed.

INVENTORY CONTROL

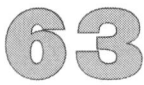

How can we manage inventory tightly but avoid running out of items?

Balancing tight inventory management and not running out of items is another challenge for many practices. The first step is to evaluate your order/sales history. Start by using your practice management software to identify items that account for the top 20 percent of product sales. Use this information to establish reorder points and reorder quantities. In most cases, inventory should turn over between every two weeks for diets to every four weeks for all other products. By establishing and following these reorder points and reorder quantities, you should always have a safety stock on hand, but never have an excess.

Most, if not all, practice management software systems include inventory modules. It should be relatively easy to set up your reorder points to print a weekly report that alerts the inventory manager to the need to reorder. Another option is to use a tag system and manage this aspect of inventory by hand.

Setting up, maintaining, and monitoring an inventory system is not an exact science—it will vary from one practice to another. A system must be reexamined on a regular basis to address changes in the general economy, seasonality of products, and unexpected occurrences.

In an ideal world a practice never runs out of a product. But the reality is it will happen, even with a good inventory management system in place. It happens, and when it does you will need to have a contingency plan in place. One possible contingency plan is to have an arrangement in place with a neighboring practice to buy or borrow products when you run out. Always have a trained second-in-command inventory person who knows the system and can monitor inventory in the absence of the primary inventory manager.

The best system will always have a way to handle the "what-ifs." In developing your inventory management system, plan and train for these scenarios.

In the near future, it may be possible to give some vendors access to your inventory module so they can resupply tomorrow what was used yesterday.

INVENTORY CONTROL

What internal controls should be in place for ordering, receiving, and dispensing inventory?

Effective inventory management includes having internal controls in place for ordering, receiving, and dispensing inventory. The person responsible for inventory management should create specific protocols for ordering, receiving, and dispensing product, with checks and balances built into the system.

Internal controls start with a preferred method for acquiring a list of needed products. This can be retrieved from the practice management system, a tag system, or zone counts. The method used depends on the experience of the inventory manager, the efficiency of the staff, and the philosophy of the practice.

Developing and using purchase orders is another excellent control measure. Purchase orders document product, size/unit, and quantity ordered and are the basis for ensuring that what was ordered did, in fact, arrive. Most practice management software systems have templates for purchase orders. If the software is set up and working properly, a purchase order can be printed with the appropriate information based on predetermined reorder points.

Upon arrival of a shipment, cross-check packing slips with the contents of the shipment and the purchase order. Ideally, someone other than the person ordering the product should perform these duties as another control measure. The person who checks in the shipment must initial the invoice or packing slip.

Staple together the purchase orders and packing slips so they can be checked with the invoice or vendor statement for accuracy. This will keep vendors honest and ensure that the practice is paying for products ordered at agreed prices.

The protocol for dispensing items must be in writing and must be announced to the staff. Client invoices must be reviewed daily for completeness and accuracy, including comparing medical records with invoices to ensure that all products and services are recorded in both places. When problems surface, having performed the medical record audit will make it easier to correct or resolve inaccuracies right away, when it's easy to recall the details of an order.

Are there items (e.g., white goods) that we do not need to track? What should be tracked most carefully (besides controlled drugs)?

Some items used by a veterinary practice are less expensive than others, and technically may not need to be tracked as carefully, but the ideal is to apply the same inventory management principles and systems to all items—inventory is money.

Most practices do not track white goods as closely as other products. The practice should identify its list of "A" (high-use or high-dollar producing) items needed on hand at all times. These "A" products vary from practice to practice. In an emergency care practice, fluids may be a high-priority product; in a general practice, heartworm and flea products may be extremely important. Other products are still important and represent monies that should be managed effectively. Everything should be tracked, even if not to the same extent as "A" items.

Though most white goods can be tracked weekly by performing visual counts, there is still value in having predetermined reorder points for these products. It is also good inventory practice to always check the pricing for these products against the previous order to ensure proper charging.

How can we adjust for seasonal trends?

Inventory should be adjusted to respond to seasonal trends. Experience will help with approximating seasonal reorder points, but you can make this more efficient and effective by using your inventory management system to track each year's trends for the same time period. Tracking trends will tell you when to add more of certain products, based on anticipated increases in business for the coming year. Reviewing reports from your practice management software, purchase orders, or vendor invoices from previous years, also helps to determine product usage history and aid in setting reorder points.

Adjusting is easy if you have adequate information. Do not be afraid to reset reorder points based on the seasonality of products (see Question 7). Create a tickler file in the inventory management program to remind you to check and adjust these points as needed. Use the program to track changes in clients' buying habits.

Always have a plan B for emergencies, such as a great working relationship with a neighboring practice, in case your practice runs out of product.

▶ Do It Now

Print a usage report for at least one typical seasonal product, such as heartworm medicine, by month for the past two years. This demonstrates whether there are seasonal fluctuations for such products and lets you adjust reorder points based on the facts.

INVENTORY CONTROL

In light of rising theft concerns, how often should we perform a physical inventory of high-dollar items?

Unfortunately but not surprisingly, high-dollar items are tempting targets for theft, which means they must be tracked and accounted for regularly. Shrinkage due to theft is controllable if the practice has adequate checks and balances.

Control measures to monitor high-dollar items for shrinkage will depend on the practice setup and philosophy. A practice with a locked central pharmacy or storage area for these products will need to perform physical counts less frequently than a practice that does not have such physical controls over its high-dollar products. Even in this scenario, however, all flats must be numbered and removed from the storage area in sequential order. This makes it easier to pinpoint, investigate, and resolve any discrepancies.

High-dollar items are commonly checked every two weeks, although some practices do so on a weekly basis. Compare the product on hand with daily invoices to check for variances. If variances appear, investigate why they occurred and correct the problem immediately. Frequency of counts should be based on past experience and the protocol established by the inventory manager.

⮕ Do It Now

To establish controls for high-dollar or high-volume items, number flats of those products and establish a written protocol to use the flats in numerical order.

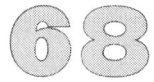

What is the best thing to do if you think product was stolen but have no idea who did it?

This is one of the most delicate challenges for the person who handles inventory management for a veterinary practice. There often is no way to identify the reason for a loss or, in the instance of employee theft, the person responsible for it, because no system for preventing shrinkage or theft is foolproof.

Locked storage areas are less vulnerable to theft than open areas to which anyone has easy access, but even locked spaces can be vulnerable to theft.

In developing an inventory program, methods specifically aimed at reducing shrinkage must be incorporated into checks and balances built into the system, to make it harder for anyone to steal products. Preventive measures start with a defined system or protocol for ordering, storing, invoicing, and taking physical counts of products.

Concentrate security efforts on high-ticket items. Start by locking up excess stock of monthly products. Allow only certain staff to have access to the storage area. Create a method for checking products out of the storage area, such as the use of written forms.

If apparent theft continues, install a video camera to monitor access to the relevant areas. Be sure to notify staff that this is being done.

Frequently perform physical counts to ensure that all products are accounted for. Do not assume that each box contains the correct number of products or vials.

There are ways to pinpoint a culprit. Theft is often committed by an employee who feels slighted in some way. Treating all employees fairly and equally can play a major role in heading off theft. Remember, desperate people do desperate things, so be aware of employees whose personal finances are not supporting their lifestyle.

If you begin to notice discrepancies, determine when they occur and who has access to the products at those times. Most theft occurs

INVENTORY CONTROL

at night when it is quiet and there is less likelihood of being discovered. If appropriate, check security access codes for the building to see whether a pattern develops between occurrences of theft and when a particular staff member accesses the building. To protect both the practice and the inventory manager's personal safety, do not attempt to apprehend anyone in the act of committing theft.

Consider posting a notice that theft is occurring but that no legal action will be taken at this point if the product is returned or replaced, and that a more vigorous inventory system will be implemented in response.

INVENTORY CONTROL

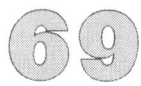

When unexplainable shortages occur, how much responsibility does the staff bear, and should any disciplinary measures be taken?

It can be difficult to assign responsibility to staff for unexplainable shortages, but disciplinary measures may be taken to eliminate such problems if an employee is identified as the culprit. Whenever there is a shortage or product, it must be investigated to identify the cause so that it can be corrected.

Consult with the practice owner or manager to develop a protocol for monitoring shrinkage and a policy for responding to shortages. The practice should have an employee handbook that details disciplinary actions that may be taken in response to carelessness, failure to follow inventory management processes, and theft. Make theft grounds for dismissal by putting this policy in your practice's employee handbook and relaying the information to all staff, initially when they join the practice and sign a statement that they have read and understand the handbook, and occasionally as a reminder.

The inventory manager is responsible for using the inventory management program to perform medical-record audits, to ensure that products are accounted for both on the medical record and in the client invoice. Consider monitoring these items on a daily basis. Suggest to the owner or manager of the practice that one person be designated to audit medical records against client invoices, checking for missed charges and making corrections as needed to ensure that both are accurate.

Awareness on everyone's part will aid in reducing shrinkage. Make it everyone's business to care about shrinkage by educating staff about how shrinkage affects the bottom line of the practice, including employee benefits, such as salary levels and raises or bonuses. But also make the staff part of the solution: Create a contest to

INVENTORY CONTROL

find and reduce missing charges; offer a prize to the department or area that makes the fewest mistakes.

If monitoring reveals that certain individuals are major repeat offenders, ask the practice owner or manager to discuss the problem with those individuals. Each incident should be documented and signed by the owner/manager and the employee involved.

⇒ Do It Now

Review your employee handbook regarding how theft is handled in your practice. If there is no section on theft, write a procedure for dealing with this issue. If there is but it is weak, seek assistance from the practice owner to strengthen it. Have this reviewed by the practice's attorney.

70

What are the best ways to deal with product and medication back orders?

Dealing with product and medication back orders is another challeging aspect of inventory management. Start by checking with alternate manufacturers or distributors to see whether they have the products, and if they do, purchase enough to cover your needs until the back order arrives. Consider a substitute, such as a chewable instead of nonchewable product, a different brand, a compounding pharmacy, or colleagues who might be able to spare an emergency supply of the product.

Set up a whiteboard in the pharmacy area to list back-ordered drugs, so the staff knows what is unavailable and when it is expected to arrive.

Make sure your vendors keep you in the loop on back orders. If you know in advance about potential reduced supplies of a product, consider acquiring a larger supply to get through the projected shortfall. Treat the acquisition as you would a bulk purchase and evaluate the pluses and minuses of buying a larger-than-usual quantity. If the numbers, cost, and billing are not suitable, it may be best to find a comparable new product instead of purchasing a large quantity.

Communication is the key. Staff, especially the doctors, must be aware of the back order so they can determine whether an alternate product will work for the present or future. Asking vendors to communicate regularly about future availability of a product will be a good test of your relationship with those vendors.

INVENTORY CONTROL

71

What should we do if inventory is missing?

When inventory is missing, the inventory manager should research which items are not accounted for and try to find out why. The reason may be a problem with the tracking system. Or, it might be someone who is lagging behind on data entry or record keeping. Because inventory discrepancies often occur for administrative or procedural reasons, it is always a good idea to consider troubleshooting steps before adjusting the numbers, since the latter will fix the count but not solve the problem.

It might be worthwhile to suggest that the practice owner, manager, or inventory manager set up a program to check for all types of shrinkage and try to identify where or how the problem occurred. Such a program would entail making adjustments until the next check, and to make the checks fairly close together—the longer the period between checks for shrinkage, the harder it will be to identify problems. Monitoring shrinkage is another reason to perform cycle counts at least monthly, when missing inventory is still fresh on everyone's mind. Present the results of these checks to owners and practice managers as regular updates on missing product and dollars lost so there are no surprises at the end of the year.

Though the inventory manager is responsible for accurate counts, practices may distribute the responsibility equally among staff. For instance, a goal of reducing inventory loss can be included as a factor in employee performance reviews. Veterinarians and owners would have to remind staff that shrinkage affects their compensation.

The owner or practice manager should ask employees to help figure out how to stop the problem and improve inventory control, again presenting the issue in terms of its effect on all employees. This will continually emphasize that inventory is everyone's responsibility.

Another approach is to set up goals of inventory accuracy levels and reward staff members for entering the appropriate information onto client invoices. If the same person is consistently responsible for discounting or missing charges, ask the practice owner or manager, or human resource manager if you have one, to discuss the issue and warn the person that he or she will be written up and disciplined according to practice policy.

If the practice has a policy on deducting inventory shrinkage from bonuses, apply it, being sure to communicate the policy when it is about to be implemented. Check with the practice's attorney to determine any legal issues to address when adhering to this type of policy. When as many of the variances as possible are resolved, make the appropriate adjustments to the inventory management program.

INVENTORY CONTROL

72

What should be in place to prevent inventory fraud?

Preventing inventory fraud is a challenge, but an inventory management system with checks and balances at all stages of the process makes it very difficult for anyone to commit inventory fraud.

One check and balance is having one individual be responsible for ordering and for a different person to receive and unpack the orders when they arrive, comparing the packing slip with the items and purchase order for accuracy. If possible, a third person should compare the purchase order and packing slip against the vendor invoice and bill. The inventory manager then enters the data on those products. This will aid in reducing the initial area of shrinkage.

Storing products—at least high-value items such as monthly heartworm and flea/tick products—in a central locked area, with a limited number of people having keys, will enhance efforts to reduce inventory fraud. Number the flats and transfer them from storage to hospital use in sequential order, which makes it easier to track them. Then use a requisition sheet to transfer to shelves for use.

Perform both regular and random inventory cycle counts. Train staff about the delicate balance between a properly functioning inventory system and clinical use of inventory products.

Missed charges can be considered as another form of theft. Performing medical-record audits of practice medical records and corresponding client invoices can help in locating missed charges so they can be reentered correctly. Audits also can reveal patterns by person, time of day, or specific products or services not being charged out properly.

INVENTORY CONTROL

73

Is it best to rotate inventory takers or to have a specific person or team in charge?

Whether it is better to rotate inventory takers or have a specific person or team in charge of inventory depends on the system your practice uses for inventory control, the size of the practice, and how many staff are available for a rotation. If this task is a one-person job, then random checks by the owner or practice manager are a good idea, because having one person responsible for ordering, unpacking, storing, and entering the data into the inventory management program does not give an inventory system adequate checks and balances.

With a team approach to taking inventory, it is also a good idea to implement random inventory checks by the owner or practice manager, because team members may not want to report colleagues who they think are stealing or misrecording inventory. Furthermore—and difficult as it may be to accept such behavior at one's veterinary practice—sometimes teams work together to commit fraud.

When considering which approach to adopt, keep in mind that rotating inventory takers can be problematic because it affects consistency, and consistency is a plus in inventory management. Suggest that the practice owner or manager designate an inventory manager and a team to assist in the process and provide the checks and balances needed to protect against fraud or theft. Not only will creating a series of quality checks save the practice money, but it will also make the staff more successful in their efforts to serve the needs of the patients.

CHAPTER 8: PRACTICE MANAGEMENT SOFTWARE

74

How do we create an inventory budget?

Having an inventory budget will make it much easier to manage inventory as the important asset it is. On an annual basis, the inventory manager should set up a budget for drugs and medical supplies. Arriving at this figure involves evaluating a combination of resources: usage reports from the previous year, projected gross for the practice, new services to be instituted, additional products that may be needed, services or products to be discontinued, and the most current benchmark (i.e., 15 percent for 2009) for drugs and medical supplies.

The practice's income statement for the previous year will have the cost of goods sold (COGS), and included within that expense category will be drugs and medical supplies. This is the dollars spent on drugs and medical supplies in that year. Use this number as the starting point for creating your budget.

Use the inventory management program to generate reports identifying usage for the year and by month. Begin by using published inventory benchmarks and aim to improve on them to create specific benchmarks for your practice.

An inventory budget is dynamic and should be reviewed and revised as needed. After all, budgets are of little help unless the practice takes the time to use the information and discover why variances and, conversely, successes occur.

75

How can we ensure that drug labels have current dates?

One aspect of inventory management is to keep only currently dated drugs in stock, which means monitoring drug expiration dates. Accurate monitoring begins with entering all drug information, including expiration dates, in the appropriate fields in the inventory module of the practice management software.

As your practice receives items from vendors, lot and expiration dates must be entered along with other relevant information. Rotation of products on the shelves (older products to the front, newer products to the back) should match the entries in the computer system, which should ensure that labels have correct dates and lot numbers for compliance purposes.

On a weekly basis, the inventory manager should perform a visual check of products and look at the expiration dates of products on the shelves. This will indicate when products are scheduled to expire so they can be used immediately, and when it might be time to return items for credit or exchange to the appropriate vendor. If there is a short-dated product, put a clearly visible warning sticker on it, to make sure it is used immediately or sent back to the vendor for credit.

76

Is there a way to track short-dated products or expiration dates that does not take a lot of time?

It may seem that tracking short-dated products or expiration dates would be time-consuming, but that is not necessarily the case. If the person responsible for inventory management makes a point of entering drug expiration dates as a matter of process, tracking becomes almost automatic. It then becomes easy to generate a list of drugs that are due to expire soon. Depending on vendor return policies, it might be a good idea to pull and replace these items or use them immediately. This will help significantly in reducing losses.

Make it part of the overall inventory management program to rotate stock and place soon-to-expire products at the front of the shelf to be used first. Suggest to the practice owner or manager that staff be trained on the importance of using these products first. A color-coded dot or tag system can alert staff, or a caution sticker or a note on the bottle highlighting the expiration date. In a weekly zone count, the zone manager can rotate stock with short-dated products to the front or mark them for return to the vendor. If problems with expiration dates are common, reorder points and reorder quantities may need to be adjusted.

Using the inventory management system to double-check orders and expiration dates can call attention to items that have been shipped in error; vendors may mistakenly send short-dated products that, if found in the unpacking process, can be sent back for credit and a longer-dated product shipped to the practice.

On the horizon is new technology that should make it easier to track expiration dates. Newer scanning systems will combine scanning and data entry via the UPC, the barcode on the product, which will reduce the time needed for data entry. At the time of sale, the scanning system will apply the appropriate information to a label and reduce inventory by the appropriate amount, which will expedite the entire process of entering and tracking product.

It is essential that the person responsible for inventory management be aware of expiration dates. The practice owner or manager should establish a protocol for ensuring that expiration dates are entered and used properly. Until more sophisticated scanners are available, accurate data entry and physically checking products on the shelves are the key to compliance and preventing shrinkage.

77

What is the best way to track in-house use of supplies (e.g., gauze, syringes)?

It can be difficult to track in-house supplies, such as gauze and syringes, that are in constant use. One way to track these items is to create a central pharmacy, either by using the inventory management system or a designated locked area in the facility. Create a sign-out sheet for syringes and white goods for designated departments as needed. This will help the inventory manager accurately track use, so that new supplies can be ordered and available when needed.

A similar approach can be taken with inventory modules in certain practice management systems, which the inventory manager can use to set up accounts such as "hospital use" for each department where the goods are used.

A zone system is another option. Each zone manager reports to the inventory manager weekly, using a spreadsheet with actual counts of products on hand. Products needed are either restocked from the central pharmacy or ordered and replaced as soon as possible. The spreadsheets will help the inventory manager track products, replace needed stock, and establish reorder points for other items.

78

How do we price critical drugs that are rarely used but needed in stock, only to expire?

Veterinary practices often keep rarely used drugs in inventory, but find that pricing these items is problematic. The question is whether the practice can break even on the cost or possibly make a small profit on such items.

The practice could charge the entire cost of the product to the first client who uses it. This at least covers the product cost and allows any future sales to become the profit.

Another suggestion is to mark up the product by 200 percent plus a higher dispensing fee. The cost of the product may be covered sooner than with typical markups.

A third approach is to merely mark it up with the same formula used for all other products and consider any loss the cost of doing business. If the product expires before it can be used or sold, the goodwill created by having it for the client at a fair price may be worthwhile.

It might be a good idea to ask the practice owner or manager to check with the doctors about whether writing a script is the better choice for such products. Sometimes stocking such a product, even though it may expire before being used, "feels right" for the doctors. If they can be educated about the associated cost and waste, they might rethink the need. At other times it may be more appropriate to partner with another local practice, and if a few drugs with the potential to expire are in stock, then maybe one practice can stock one product and the other practice can stock the other product, allowing for borrowing when needed.

Look at the mission statement of the practice and see whether it aids in making the decision. Once the decision has been made, put the protocol in writing and disseminate it throughout the practice so everyone knows how to handle this situation in the future.

79

Rarely used medications are often thrown away at expiration. Is there a better way to track medications that will soon expire?

Because rarely used medications are often thrown out when they expire, they represent wasted money as well as product loss, making it even more important to track expiration dates. One of the best ways to handle this problem is to track the expiration dates on products. This can be done by marking the bottles or using colored sticky notes with the expiration date. Once the bottles are marked, they need to be checked on a weekly basis. If any expiration date is within the next three months, these bottles need to be placed at the front of the cabinet for immediate use. At the same time, the staff needs to be informed of the list of products with short dating. This can be done by a memo, posting of a list, or at the next scheduled client service meeting with an announcement regarding the list of short-dated products. The more you can inform the staff, the more likely they will use the products before they expire.

If your practice management software tracks these dates, make sure this information is entered at the time of receiving the product. On a quarterly basis, run a "look forward" report on which products will be expiring in the next quarter and act appropriately to use the products.

If you find medications near expiration, you will need to examine why it is happening. Is it because of short expiration dates from the last order? Another reason could be ordering too much of the product. Turns of 10 to 12 times a year should be the goal for most practices.

If you have products that are extremely close to expiration contact your supplier to see if you can return and exchange the product or receive a credit. If the product has expired, be sure to review your

OSHA handbook for the best method of disposing of it; it may not be wise to simply throw it out. Regularly throwing away expired products is costly. Make every effort to reduce shrinkage to avoid losing money.

➡ Do It Now

Check your practice management software to see if there is a "look forward" report. If not, call the software support service and have them guide you in setting it up so you can easily track expiring medications.

How do we use software for inventory recording and monitoring?

Persuading the practice owner or manager, and other staff to use the software programs available for recording and monitoring inventory can be tricky. Some people are computer-phobic and resist using inventory management programs. Others are more comfortable with programs but not using them to their full potential.

The first step is usually to educate the owner or manager about what such programs can do—that they can make it easier and more efficient to keep track of products and supplies that everyone needs and uses, which will save money. If the owner or manager is already on board, the next step is to educate staff and reassure everyone that inventory management is not intended to replace people but to make their jobs easier.

Most, if not all, practice management software systems have an integrated inventory program; some of these programs are very user-friendly. They can provide an immense amount of information more efficiently than tracking by hand. In addition to tracking usage of products and integrating with client invoicing, other, often underused, tasks of these programs include setting up reorder points for products, creating purchase orders, tracking expiration dates for products, managing total dollar value of inventory, and tracking controlled substances. It requires time and energy to learn about, set up, and make the most of a practice inventory management program, but it is worth the effort.

Take a few days to explore the software to discover its capabilities. Ask tech support if advanced training on the inventory module is available. If so, the inventory manager should take such training.

Consider creating or joining a software user group to share mentorship among other veterinary practices using the same program.

PRACTICE MANAGEMENT SOFTWARE

There probably are a number of inventory managers who would enjoy discussing issues and solutions. Rather than wait for someone else to take action, make some calls and start a local users' group.

81

How can we trust in the accuracy of our computerized inventory numbers?

It can be difficult to trust the accuracy of a computerized inventory management system, especially if it is new to the veterinary practice. The key to reliability is to enter accurate information and manage it effectively. Human error tends to create many of the problems associated with accuracy of computerized inventory management. The only way to trust the accuracy of your computer inventory numbers is to create a workable system and train everyone to use it properly.

This is why implementing both formal protocols or processes and a series of checks and balances is vital if the system is to reflect a count closer to actual inventory. How the practice tracks in-house use of products, injectables, or invoice entry errors plays a key role in the accuracy of the system. Encourage staff to participate in entering or recording information at every point in practice activities. Make it easier for staff to do their part, and reward them for doing so.

A combination of cycle counts (counting "A" products monthly, "B" products every other month, and everything else once a quarter), medical-record audits (comparing medical records with client invoices for accuracy of both), and reviewing quantities on hand (checking computer inventory quantities against visual counts for accuracy) will help.

Barcoding and scanning items at the time they are added to inventory, and at the time of use, will improve accuracy in tracking product. Use of this technology in the veterinary industry is still in its infancy, but as it becomes more common, inventory accuracy will improve greatly.

82

How is it possible to get every inventory item in the computer for inventory (e.g., syringe use, vet wrap)?

Getting every inventory item into the computer is, indeed, a challenge. It takes time and energy to enter the information. If the inventory manager makes it easy and essentially automatic to enter the information, it will become less difficult.

One option is to set up surgery, outpatient pharmacy, and treatment as clients in the inventory management system, with items like tape, bandage material, and syringes dispensed as whole units (boxes, not individual rolls or syringes) to those areas. That way, inventory can be counted out from one central stockroom (in the computer or a central location). Once something leaves the stockroom, it should be moved in the inventory management program as well (i.e., surgery, treatment, outpatient pharmacy, and so on). This helps with keeping reorder points for these items in the computer and then maintaining their accuracy.

With most practice's margins being squeezed by other retailers, it is paramount to make the time to enter this information and then use it. Knowing the cost and use of syringes, for instance, helps with determining better pricing for services and negotiating new prices with vendors. The savings in time, energy, and costs are worth the effort.

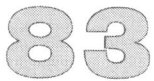

How do you use the computer more efficiently for inventory management, such as printing reports and obtaining statistics?

The computer can make aspects of inventory management such as these more efficient. If a veterinary practice is using a practice inventory management program only for invoicing, it is not making maximum use of the program's capabilities.

The first step is for the inventory manager to seek resources to improve understanding of the program. This can be accomplished by reading the software manual, exploring the program, contacting technical support, attending user meetings, or befriending another user. The more you know about what the program can do, the better use you can make of it. It may be necessary to ask the practice owner or manager to give the inventory manager time and support for additional training.

One way to make more and better use of the system is to review the selection of reports relating to inventory by looking at where the numbers come from and what the report is attempting to tell you. Some reports will help set reorder points, while others may track expiring drugs. The reports will identify information from different areas of the inventory and help you manage inventory better. Print out reports on a regular basis to share with appropriate colleagues throughout the veterinary practice, from the owner or manager to the receptionist at the front desk, so everyone can see what is going on with inventory and get a sense of their role in improving control and cost-effectiveness.

Combining report functions with better use of inventory module software will enhance inventory management skills. Understanding the program's capabilities will help the inventory manager create a better inventory management system.

PRACTICE MANAGEMENT SOFTWARE

⏵ Do It Now

Go to the report module, investigate the entire list of preinstalled report templates, and determine which ones will work for your practice. If you do not find one, call technical support and ask for help in setting up the reports or templates needed to manage inventory for the practice.

PRACTICE MANAGEMENT SOFTWARE

How do we get accurate inventory counts if we do not have a central storage area under lock and key?

Achieving and maintaining accurate inventory counts can be difficult in a practice that does not have a central storage area under lock and key. This is where an inventory management program becomes essential. The likelihood of computer quantities and shelf counts being accurate for longer than a day is minimal. The goal is to reduce human error while keeping both computer quantities and physical counts as close and accurate as possible.

If you do not have a designated central storage area, use a closet with a lockable door to store and manage high-dollar inventory items. If that is not possible, suggest that the owner or manager purchase a key-locked storage cabinet and find a safe place for it. Even a small lockable cabinet can hold high-dollar, fast-turning products that are valuable both to the practice and on the street. Protecting those items is an investment in the financial well-being of the practice.

Even without a locked, central storage area, the inventory manager should take a look at all aspects of the inventory management system to determine how to create a strategy to control inventory that includes the ordering process, data entry, invoicing, and monitoring for accuracy while reducing shrinkage.

Start by looking at each piece of the inventory puzzle to determine which areas work and which areas need help. Strategize ways to correct any weaknesses or inefficient processes. Seek advice from peers and colleagues in user groups and at other practices. Look at the manual and e-bulletins from your software vendor.

Once a new process is developed and ready for implementation, have the staff review it to ensure they understand it, and be sure to explain the value of adding it to the practice's protocols. Also be sure to make staff training part of the process, and include the doctors in the training, since they too work with inventory. Each area of the practice may have certain people who need training.

Once everyone is trained, implement the program and reevaluate it in 60 to 90 days. At that time, make adjustments if necessary. Change is difficult—be patient.

CHAPTER 9: CONTROLLED SUBSTANCES AND INJECTABLES

What is the best way to handle controlled drug inventory (i.e., how much of each drug is appropriate to have in stock in the safe)?

Handling controlled drug inventory and determining how much of each drug should be kept in stock are vital. The first objective is to make sure the veterinary practice follows all guidelines for managing controlled substances as defined on the Drug Enforcement Administration's (DEA) website. Make sure you have the proper paperwork for recording acquired products and documenting usage, starting with a log for controlled substances. Logs are essential for tracking usage as well as for completing the paper trail needed for compliance issues.

Use the practice management software to track usage and determine the amount and frequency of orders. Have a secondary method of tracking usage and quantities on hand—a physical count, which can be daily, weekly, or monthly, depending on the needs of the veterinary practice—as a checks-and-balances system to ensure more accurate tracking of these products.

Regularly—ideally, weekly—monitor logs, inventory counts, and medical records for accuracy. If discrepancies arise, they must be examined and corrected immediately. If frequency or character of discrepancies continues, reexamine protocols and make changes to ensure better compliance with the law.

All controlled substances must be under lock and key, and access to the products should be limited to appropriate personnel, such as doctors and one other reliable person. To protect these products from theft, consider installing a video camera with continuous recording in or aimed at the locked storage area.

There is no surefire, one-size-fits-all way to manage controlled substances. So long as human beings must log items into and out of

CONTROLLED SUBSTANCES AND INJECTABLES

the system, there will always be a risk of errors and shrinkage. It is best to be highly concerned about accuracy and continually compare logs with physical counts. Make sure all employees know that there are legal consequences, including substantial fines, that could shut down a practice for failing to manage inventory of controlled substances.

CONTROLLED SUBSTANCES AND INJECTABLES

What are the protocols for controlled substances?

Protocols for controlled substances originate from various federal and state agencies. The practice owner or manager should have knowledge of these protocols as well as a current DEA registration number approved for scheduled products used in the veterinary practice.

All appropriate forms for ordering product must be current and kept under lock and key. Make sure that staff know and follow the practice's approved guidelines for documenting proof of ordering and receipt of these products. At least annually, review the requirements for ordering and maintaining controlled substances. Be sure to create a protocol that incorporates all of this important information and to share throughout the practice.

Controlled substances must be kept separate from other drugs in a secure, locked cabinet. A designated individual should check all products received against order forms for accuracy. The order form should be initialed and dated by the person receiving the order, in order to document that the product was received. Each vial must be coded or labeled according to established protocols, for both legal and accounting purposes, and used in sequential order.

Use of controlled substances must be properly documented in a controlled substance log that is maintained consistently. Only certified personnel should be allowed access to where items are secured or to record movement of items in the controlled substance log.

Controlled substances must be monitored on a weekly basis, through inventory counts, to make sure all products are accounted for, and then compared with the log. A medical record audit comparing the log with client invoices and medical records must be included in the protocol. This will ensure that the inventory manager can account for the product on client invoices, medical records, and the log.

CONTROLLED SUBSTANCES AND INJECTABLES

What do we do with expired controlled substances?

Disposing of controlled substances has legal and environmental consequences; these items cannot simply be tossed into the trash. Check with your state regulatory agency to determine the approved method for disposal of expired controlled substances. If your state does not have rules, then you must follow federal guidelines for disposal. The agency—state or federal—with the strictest set of rules governing controlled substances is the one to follow. In general, either agency will require that the practice keep a log of these items that shows when they expired and how they were disposed of. In some states, approved biohazard containers may be used, while others require that specific government agencies handle disposal, or that a reverse distributor does. Do not flush the product down the drain. There is growing ecological concern about pharmaceutical products contaminating water sources.

Make sure the practice has a written policy regarding all aspects of proper disposal of expired controlled substances, which all staff have read and signed, and that it is followed fully and consistently. Documentation of disposal is essential for compliance with the law—it also protects the veterinary practice from damaging fines.

⇒ Do It Now

Locate your state's Practice Act and read the section on controlled substances. If you are unable to find one in the general files, ask the medical director or owner of the practice for his or her copy. If no one can provide a copy, contact your state veterinary medical board or your state controlled substance agency and request a copy immediately. Become familiar with the guidelines and create a policy for disposing of expired controlled substances so that the practice is in compliance with all aspects of the Controlled Substance Act.

What controlled substance checks help keep logs and inventory accurate?

The inventory manager can use several checks to keep logs and inventory of controlled substances accurate.

The best way to maintain an accurate controlled substance log is to monitor the log itself, compare it with a physical count of the products, and regularly update the computer inventory levels of those products. Frequency may vary with the type of veterinary practice—an emergency/critical care practice may monitor controlled substances at the end of each shift, while a general companion animal practice may check quantities only weekly or monthly.

Limit the number of people with access to the locked are used to store controlled substances. If the practice has a locked and limited-access storage area for these and transfers items to a locked treatment cabinet, make sure such transfers can be made only by prior authorization, with a sign-out form and formal transfer process. Aim for a system that incorporates a well-documented paper trail.

Who is qualified to write controlled drug prescriptions?

Veterinarians are the only ones who can prescribe controlled substances, but each state has its own guidelines as to who can administer them. In most states, anyone the veterinarian feels is qualified to administer these products is allowed to do so, as long as a licensed veterinarian is supervising.

In most practices, a certified, licensed, or registered veterinary technician administers these products. These technicians are trained, during their formal schooling, on the importance of maintaining accurate records for such products and are the logical first choice for this task. However, they still will be under the supervision of a veterinarian.

The practice should establish a policy designating who is to administer these products. This means creating and relaying a complete training program regarding controlled substance protocols that addresses who has the keys to the lockbox, where the logs are kept, who keeps them up-to-date, and how products are tracked from arrival to final deposition. The entire process has to follow the letter of the law and the policies of the practice.

How many staff members should handle controlled drugs?

Determining who should handle controlled drugs is fairly easy: as few as possible. If your veterinary practice has a small staff, only one or two staff members, plus each doctor, should have a role in administering controlled substances. For larger facilities, a larger number of qualified staff (veterinary technicians, for example) may have access to controlled substances, provided all have had training in their handling and care. It is wise to set up a schedule that designates which staff members are responsible for controlled substances (either for a day or for a shift) to ensure better compliance.

The people holding the keys must be responsible for knowing and understanding the protocols for controlled substances to ensure compliance and accurate tracking of these items. Management's responsibility is to ensure that complete and proper training in handling controlled substances is made available to these individuals.

Most practices assign two team members to handle controlled substances at any one time. This could be a veterinarian and one other qualified staff person per shift, such as a veterinary technician. These persons should have keys to the controlled substance cabinet in their possession during their shift. They are responsible for logging in the appropriate information for tracking purposes and for performing a physical count of all controlled substances at the end of the shift.

Reducing the number of people with access to the controlled substance cabinet makes it easier to monitor the cabinet and ensure the accuracy of logs.

CONTROLLED SUBSTANCES AND INJECTABLES

91

How can we keep better inventory on injectable drugs?

Every veterinary practice must keep accurate inventory records on its injectable drugs. One of the first criteria to be decided is how use of the product will be tracked. This is where practice management software becomes valuable. Start by entering the product when it arrives and use milliliter (ml) as the dispensing quantity; then add an injection charge, similar to a dispensing fee, to the item cost. This process allows the inventory manager and the practice management software to track the quantity used and know when to reorder. Recording quantities used on the client invoice is vital to an accurate count.

Consider identifying one member of the practice team to review medical records, travel sheets, and invoices for inconsistency on a regular basis. For example, if the injectable drug is used on a hospitalized patient, the quantity used can be properly entered in all documents before the patient is discharged. If it is used on an outpatient, it may be discovered at a later date; it can still be corrected and properly recorded. This system may identify problems in entering products into the inventory module or in charting services, or with individuals who are consistently forgetting to record entries in the medical record or invoice.

If the practice protocol is not to track each milliliter of a product in the practice management software, but to charge a set fee for an injection, then someone will have to perform a physical count of the injectable inventory. This may be done weekly, semimonthly, or monthly, or can be combined with a tag system whereby the reorder point tag is removed from the vial and placed in a bin for the inventory manager to add to the next order.

What can we do to prevent theft of controlled substances?

Preventing the theft of controlled substances starts with asking good questions while interviewing a candidate for employment, and following up on references. According to Section 1301.90 of the Code of Federal Regulations, it is permissible to ask potential employees the following questions:

- "Within the past three years, have you ever knowingly used any narcotics, amphetamines, or barbiturates other than those prescribed by your physician?" If someone answers "yes," ask for details and follow up on the responses.
- "Within the past five years, have you been convicted of a felony? Within the past two years, have you been charged with a misdemeanor or other criminal offense?"

The owner, manager, or human resources manager of the practice may check on whether a potential employee has a criminal record. The employment application should include the applicant's signed authorization allowing the practice to make inquiries to the courts or other law enforcement agencies. An applicant who will be working with controlled substances must execute this authorization; in most cases, this will be a veterinarian. Let the applicant know that any information furnished by the court or other agencies will not automatically prevent employment, but will be used to better evaluate the candidate for the position.

Assuming the practice has checked references and hired qualified employees to handle its controlled substances, the next step is to create a training program to ensure that controlled substances are properly monitored and accounted for. Training should start with how to use logs and other monitoring activities for controlled substances.

CONTROLLED SUBSTANCES AND INJECTABLES

Training also should emphasize that all prescription pads must be kept under lock and key to prevent theft. It is not uncommon to find prescription pads with the veterinarian's Drug Enforcement Agency number in exam room drawers. They should be kept in a locked, secure controlled substance box.

Daily counts of products and comparisons with the logbook also head off theft. Tighten security measures for controlled substances as discussed in previous questions. Ensure that all staff understand that theft is grounds for dismissal. Put this in writing and remind staff of it regularly.

⇒ Do It Now

Review your interview questions for hiring applicants who may be asked to fill a script for a controlled substance. If the questions above are not in your list, add them. Include checking references as part of the preemployment process.

93

Should we be charging for injectable drugs by the milliliter instead of using a flat injection fee?

Injectable drugs can be priced by the milliliter used or at a flat fee, or a combination of the two. The choice depends on which method best fits into the practice's inventory management. If managing inventory is a priority, the use of a per milliliter plus an injection fee is the best choice and appears to be the overwhelming choice of respondents to a 2009 AAHA inventory survey.

A flat fee can be effective but makes more work for the inventory manager in maintaining proper levels of injectable products—he or she will need to revisit the inventory module daily and adjust the quantity on hand regularly to keep the information up-to-date and accurate.

Holding frank and honest discussions with the veterinarians and technical staff can resolve this issue. If a flat fee is the choice, the discussion should focus on managing injectables to maintain proper levels of product without tying up more money on the shelves than necessary. As a result, frequent monitoring of injectables will be necessary to ensure the practice does not run out of these products.

If the practice elects to track injectables per milliliter, the inventory manager will need to ensure that all the fields in the inventory module are set up to actually do so. Data entry should be performed by the same person to ensure consistency and accuracy.

CHAPTER 10: INVENTORY MANAGER CONCERNS

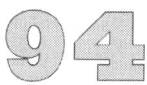

What is the best way to keep up with product turnover?

Keeping up with how much product you have left on the shelf and how frequently you run through products is an ongoing effort for any veterinary practice, but a good inventory management system and staff feedback will help. The staff must be accountable and responsible for notifying the practice manager or inventory manager when products are running low. A good tag or zone system (see Question 1) will aid in this process. Setting realistic reorder points and reorder quantities will also help. If a practice runs out of a needed item, it is time to reevaluate reorder points and reorder quantities and the inventory management system in general.

Many practice management software programs allow for tracking exactly what is in the hospital at a given time based on the last receipt date and when an item was used or was sold. If your practice isn't already using a software program in this capacity, it will take time and training to set up. But it will be worth the investment.

Determining product usage (see Questions 7 and 9) and adjusting for seasonality as needed will also help in monitoring turnover more closely, so that you do not run out of products or let them sit on the shelves for too long.

INVENTORY MANAGER CONCERNS

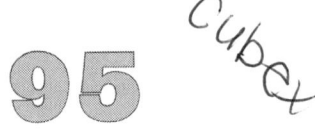

95

If we are not using a computerized inventory system, what system works best for tracking items in inventory and determining when they need to be ordered?

Some veterinary practices prefer not to use computerized inventory management systems. In those instances, a tag or card system may work well. It is tedious to use, but can be effective so long as someone is responsible for managing and maintaining it.

Start by creating a draft inventory management program and identifying the person responsible for completing and overseeing the program. Then organize the inventory and stock items by category, so it is clear where things are. Marking shelves or closets with product names also works well.

Once items are categorized and bottles are accounted for, determine reorder points. Start with an educated guess about what reorder points should be. Track usage to arrive at accurate reorder points.

Once reorder points are in place, put a tag on the reorder bottle with the product name, date ordered, vendor, and last known cost. The challenge is training staff to place the tags in a reorder basket whenever they notice the tags. Create a want list in case tags are misplaced and there is critical need for a product.

On a weekly basis, retrieve the basket contents to develop a purchase order. It is advisable to also perform a visual inspection of the products at this time. Reorder tags are frequently misplaced, but the visual inspection should catch products with inventory levels below their reorder points, so they can be added to the next order.

Develop record-keeping sheets with the names of products present and visible approximate reorder points. This will become a reminder, when doing a visual count of products, to ensure that reorder points are accurate and the practice is not running out of product.

INVENTORY MANAGER CONCERNS

With a handwritten inventory management system, it is more important than ever for the person responsible for inventory to re-educate the staff about the tag system. It will take continual training and effort by all staff members to track inventory and follow the procedure for identifying the time to reorder products.

*Weekly zone$ counts

INVENTORY MANAGER CONCERNS

96

How can we best determine a well-balanced amount of inventory to keep on hand?

To make the most of its assets, cash, products, and human resources, every veterinary practice must determine its ideal balance of inventory to keep on hand. When deciding this for your practice, you need to consider a few factors. The goal for many practices is to have $15,000 to $18,000 of inventory per doctor. Other practices promote a 30-day turnover rate for most products and do not want to have more than a 30-day supply on the shelf at any one time; setting reorder quantities to support a 30-day supply is therefore important and can be accomplished by reviewing sales and usage reports, remembering to allow for seasonal usage of some products, and factoring in delivery times. You also have to look at reorder points. Monitor these points on a regular basis to maintain the balance of product and costs, attempting to have products turn 10 to 12 times a year.

Attaining a well-balanced inventory should also involve the inventory manager working with the practice owner, manager, and doctors to eliminate duplicate medications (i.e., meds that do the same thing but include different brands preferred by different doctors). Ask the doctors to discuss and agree on a primary product and a secondary one as the backup or plan B.

Some practices have switched to weekly zone counts to reduce inventory on hand. The main advantage of this system is that it can reduce reorder points, which helps improve cash flow. Typical zones are food, outpatient pharmacy, surgical/treatment area, and receptionist area. Zones help in managing inventory, both in balancing products on hand and in cash outlay.

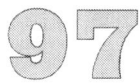

How do we know if we are managing inventory well?

There is a multitude of ways to know whether a veterinary practice is managing its inventory efficiently and effectively. One is more anecdotal than scientific: There will be fewer instances of someone saying, "We just ran out of something."

Another proof the process is working is that fewer products are expiring on the shelves and requiring disposal or return to vendors. A well-managed system makes a point of tracking expiration dates.

Results of checking the inventory turnover ratio also indicate an effective inventory management system and process. Products should turn 10 to 12 times a year; some will turn more often and others less. If the practice has met this benchmark without running out of product, the inventory management system is working. The goal is first to meet inventory benchmarks, and then to improve on them without running out of product.

Financial reports plus reports from the inventory management system should indicate whether the practice has reduced its cost of goods sold and, more important, its drugs and medical supplies; and, in turn, improved profitability through better inventory management. The goal of inventory management is to ensure that the practice has the products it needs to treat patients, for both wellness and sickness, while improving its cash flow.

Managing inventory is a matter of balancing all aspects of inventory (ordering, stocking, using, and selling) by continually monitoring and correcting when needed. Inventory management is an art that will provide opportunities for improvement. It is a moving target and always will be. Be diligent and patient in your pursuit of well-managed inventory.

INVENTORY MANAGER CONCERNS

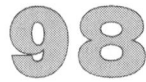

How do we fit inventory management into a busy schedule?

For many veterinary practices, it can seem almost impossible to fit inventory management into an already busy schedule. Admittedly, managing inventory successfully is a multiday task that must be a priority for the inventory manager and for the practice. Once a system is in place, though, it will be easier for the inventory manager to order and track supplies and product, enter new product information, evaluate specials, and manage other types of information that are key to a profitable practice. In addition, the inventory management system should save time rather than take up more time.

A skilled inventory manager can easily recoup his or her salary by improving inventory management. Inventory is one of the biggest expenses in any veterinary practice. If managed well, it can improve profitability.

The best use of time is to put in place a strategy to manage inventory. Break it down into bite-size pieces, rather than trying to do everything in one day. It requires time and patience to craft a strong, workable, and efficient inventory management system.

For a veterinary practice to be successful, inventory management must be a priority. This might mean hiring a new person or adjusting schedules and revamping job descriptions so a current employee can perform this task.

⇒ Do It Now

Look at current staff assignments and schedules, and delegate the tasks that do not need your full attention to someone who is capable of handling them. Managing inventory effectively is time well spent, and must be a priority.

INVENTORY MANAGER CONCERNS

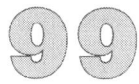

Is there a rule of thumb for a big order that we buy now and pay for later?

Many veterinary practices look for a rule of thumb for handling things like big orders that can be ordered now and paid for later, but a rule of thumb falls somewhere between a mathematical formula and a shot in the dark. That said, there are no rules of thumb for big orders. Whether to buy now and pay later for larger orders will depend on the practice and its philosophy of inventory management.

Investigate all promotions as though they were completely different. Evaluate the effect of each promotion on cash flow. If it fits your needs and storage space, pursue it. If not, say no and move on.

In evaluating the potential cost savings of a big order, look for at least a 10 percent discount for a three-month supply of product. If the appropriate quantity is purchased, delayed billing will let the practice collect payments for the product before the bill from the vendor is due. Just be sure that funds are available to pay the bill when it arrives, rather than incur interest or late charges that end up negating the savings of the bulk order.

Timing of a purchase is also a factor. Buying springtime products in the fall is not a good move. One of the reasons why vendors offer specials in the fall is to reduce their warehouse supplies and reduce the inventory tax they may incur. In some states, inventory taxes on veterinary products are due in December, and the practice may have to pay an inventory tax on those products if it buys in bulk at this time. If this is the case, try to negotiate a higher discount to cover that expense.

INVENTORY MANAGER CONCERNS

100

What do we do about the large amount of waste materials (cardboard boxes, padding, and plastic bags) associated with shipped purchases?

Every business, including a veterinary practice, ends up with a large amount of waste materials as a result of receiving vendor orders. Recycling is an excellent way to process mass packing and packaging materials. Develop a recycling program in your practice that includes these materials and go one step farther by using recycled paper for client invoices and educational material.

Some vendors recycle packing material and containers. Ask your sales reps or vendors if they have a program for reusing any part of a shipment. If so, then incorporate their program into your plan.

Some bubble wrap and packing peanuts can be reused to protect products sent to clients, when sending lab specimens to outside reference laboratories, or for in-house purposes. A local packaging store might accept the remainder of the packing material. Cardboard is easily recycled through local programs and trash pickup services.

If your practice has a recycling program, promote it in your marketing. Let your clients know they visit a "green" practice that is proud to help the environment. You can do this in newsletters, on your website, on invoices (identifying your use of recycled paper), and on labels on recycling bins for clients' trash.

101

How do you tell if a bulk buy is a good move in terms of all aspects of inventory management?

Bulk buys are tempting because they save money, but may not be a good move if they take up too much space on your shelves, do not move quickly, or tie up funds that are needed for more urgent uses. A bulk buy must be evaluated by the amount of savings offered, product already on the shelf, and time to use the product. Special financing/delayed billing can also be a consideration. The question is whether it is worth having a large amount of inventory (cash) sitting on the shelf waiting to be sold, or whether that money can be used for other purchases or investments.

There are several factors to recognize when you are approached with a "big deal." The first is how much product the veterinary practice really needs for how long. Look at deals for only your "A" products. Use the inventory management software to research usage of the product by month for the past year. This will give you an idea of quantity to order for a specific period of time. In most cases, a three-month supply is the most any practice needs—and has space to store—of any one item.

Expiration dates are also a concern with large orders. Be wary of short-dated products. In some cases, short-dating can be used as a negotiating tool to increase a discount. Just be sure everyone in the practice is aware of the date limit on the product so it is used, rather than going to waste, which again would cancel out the benefit of a big order.

Each bulk offer should be considered on the basis of three factors: whether the veterinary practice needs the product, quantity needed at any given time, and type of billing for the deal.

Assuming all three factors line up, it makes more sense to look at purchasing up to a 90-day supply of a product if the discount is

INVENTORY MANAGER CONCERNS

sufficient. The discount should be 3 to 5 percent per month's supply of the product. For a three-month supply, the discount should be 10 percent or greater.

RESOURCES

Groups and Associations

American Animal Hospital Association, Veterinary Management School (VMS), Level One (Lakewood, CO), www.aaha.org.

Center for Cognitive Liberty & Ethics, www.cognitive libery.org/statelaws.html

Drug Enforcement Administration (DEA), www.justice.gov/dea/pbubs/csa.html

Veterinary Hospital Managers Association, Inc., P.O. Box 2280, Alachua, FL 32616; www.vhma.org

Publications

Ackerman, Lowell, DVM, DACVD, MBA, MPA. *Management Basics for Veterinarians* (ASJA Press, 2003).

Ackerman, Lowell, DVM, DACVD, MBA, MPA. *Blackwell's Five-Minute Veterinary Practice Management Consult* (Blackwell Publishing, 2007).

American Animal Hospital Association. *AAHA Controlled Substance Logs*, Second Edition (AAHA Press, 2010).

Heinke, Marsha, DVM, EA, CPA, CVPM, and John B. McCarthy, DVM, MBA. *Practice Made Perfect: A Complete Guide to Veterinary Practice Management*, Second Edition (AAHA Press, 2012).

McCarthy, J. *Basic Guide to Veterinary Hospital Management*, Second Edition (American Animal Hospital Association, 1995).

Opperman, M., *The Art of Veterinary Practice Management* (Veterinary Publishing Group, 1999).

Seibert, Phillip J., Jr., CVT. *Be Safe! Manager's Guide to Hazardous Substances* (AAHA Press, 2007).

Wanamaker, B. P., DVM, MS, and K. L. Massey, LVMT. *Applied Pharmacology for Veterinary Technicians*, Fourth Edition (Saunders, 2009).

Websites

AAHA *Trends*: http://trends.aaha.org

Drug Enforcement Agency: www.justice.gov/dea/pubs/csa.html

ProxyRx: www.mwivet.com/SERVICES

Seibert, Phillip J.: www.safetyvet.com

Stericycle: Medical waste disposal guidelines, www.stericycle.com

Veterinary Economics: www.dvm360.com

Veterinary Information Network: www.vin.com

veterinarymanager.wordpress.com

RESOURCES

Webster Veterinary University, Inventory Module: www.webstervet.com
www.cognitiveliberty.org/dll/statelaws.htm
www.vetcentric.com
www.vetstreet.com

LIST OF CONTRIBUTORS

Adams, Justina, Capitol Area Animal Medical Center, Harrisburg, PA
Aitchison, Kathleen, Cape Cod Veterinary Specialists, Buzzards Bay, MA
Alimossy, Dyana, CVT, Riverside Park Veterinary Clinic, Grants Pass, OR
Arnold, Cheryl, Veterinary Medical Center, Easton, MD
Baty, Margaret, Wilderness Animal Hospital, Maple Valley, WA
Bender, Stacy, Great Bridge Veterinary Hospital, Chesapeake, VA
Bernardi, Renee, Arbor View Animal Hospital, Valparaiso, IN
Bittler, Melinda, LVT, Boulevard Animal Hospital, Richmond, VA
Brahm, Sue, CVT, Lakeside Animal Hospital, Milwaukee, WI
Brehaut, Cindy, Capeway Veterinary Hospital, Fairhaven, MA
Brown, Carmen S., Avon Lake Animal Clinic, Avon Lake, OH
Brownell, Joanne, LVT, Liverpool Village Animal Hospital, Liverpool, NY
Buhlig-Arnold, Heather, St. Charles Veterinary Clinic, St. Charles, IL
Busse, Steve, Park Centre Animal Hospital, Alameda, CA
Bynaker, Kaleen, Gaithersburg Animal Hospital, Gaithersburg, MD
Carter, Karli, Payson Family Pet Hospital, Payson, UT
Cawston, David, MHA, Back Bay Veterinary Clinic, Boston, MA
Cochrane, Heather, Urban Vet Care, Denver, CO
Cohron, Tammy, LVT, Pet Clinic PC, Omaha, NE
Collari, Cathryn, LVT, Mountain Park Animal Hospital, Lilburn, GA
Collins, Nickey, French Creek Veterinary Hospital, Pottstown, PA
Cousins, Craig, VRCC, Englewood, CO
Dawson, Cindy, Edgewood Animal Clinic, Lakeland, FL
DeDeo, Joseph, Upstate Veterinary Specialties, Latham, NY
DeGesero, Stephanie, Judge Ely Animal Hospital, Abilene, TX
DeVaul, Candace, Chittenango Animal Hospital, Chittenango, NY
Diffin, Janette, Northern Animal Clinic, Midland, MI
Douglas, Amy, Cascade Veterinary Referral Center, Portland, OR

LIST OF CONTRIBUTORS

DuBois, Carla, LVT, Chambers Creek Veterinary Hospital, Lakewood, WA
Duda, Heather, Gamble Pet Clinic, Fort Collins, CO
Dunn, Katrina, Colony Animal Hospital, Newport News, VA
Dunphy, Clyde, DVM, Capitol Illini Veterinary Services, Springfield, IL
Dzialo, Alicia, Harrison Memorial Animal Hospital, Denver, CO
Erickson, Denise, CVT, Denise, PineRidge Pet Care, Andover, MN
Ewing, Nichole, Heartwood Animal Hospital, Youngsville, NC
Felix, Janet, Quakertown Veterinary Clinic, Quakertown, PA
Fenner, Chris, RVT, Bernardo Heights Veterinary Hospital, San Diego, CA
Finnegan, Nikki, Flannery Animal Hospital, New Windsor, NY
Foreman, Terri, Southpark Veterinary Hospital, Broken Arrow, OK
Frame, Robert, Arbor Pet Hospital, Wilton Manors, FL
Frost, Nicole, CVT, Prescott Animal Hospital, Prescott, AZ
Funk, Paula, New Hope Animal Hospital, New Hope, MN
Gatz, Cindy, Broadway Veterinary Clinic, Leavenworth, KS
Geronimo, Lisa, Pearland Animal Hospital West, Pearland, TX
Gilbert, Juli, CVT, Orchard Hills Animal Hospital, Washougal, WA
Glashauser, Kelly, RVT, Midland Animal Clinic, Midland, MI
Goelz, Cathy, Animal Emergency Clinic, Greenville, SC
Goulet, Racheal, LVT, Murray Animal Hospital, Murray, KY
Graham, Rob, CVT, Animal Health Services, Cave Creek, AZ
Grittner, Renee, Pewee Valley Veterinary Center, Pewee Valley, KY
Gunnoe, Robin R., Animal Care Associates, Inc., Charleston, WV
Hammond, JoAnn, Eye Clinic Veterinary, LLC, Wheat Ridge, CO
Hanks, Becky, Ravenwood Veterinary Clinic, Port Orange, FL
Hanks, Kendra, RVT, Dakota Hills Veterinary Clinic, Rapid City, SD
Haugland, Gail, Faust Animal Hospital, Phoenix, AZ
Hawkins, David, Dogwood Pet Hospital, Gresham, OR
Hill, Julie, Jonesboro Family Pet Hospital, Jonesboro, AR
Huppert, Emily, CVT, Hudson Road Animal Hospital, Woodbury, MN
Ives, Noreen, Russell Animal Hospital, PA, Concord, NH
Jackson, Judi, Centerville Animal Hospital, Snellville, GA

LIST OF CONTRIBUTORS

Janssen, Dana, CVT, Oakwood Hills Animal Hospital, Eau Claire, WI
Jimenez, Regina, Alamo Dog & Cat Hospital, San Antonio, TX
Julia, Muller Veterinary Hospital, Walnut Creek, CA
King, Michael W., DVM, Pet Street Station Animal Hospital, Norwich, NY
Kocsis, Cathy, West Mountain Animal Hospital, Bennington, VT
Kolker, Shannon, Friendship Veterinary Hospital, Ft. Walton Beach, FL
Krueger, Danita, LVT, Temperance Animal Hospital, Temperance, MI
Lake, Vivian, RVT, Eastside Animal Hospital, Jeffersonville, IN
Lassiter, Susan, CVPM, All Creatures Animal Hospital, Dunwoody, GA
Lewis, Donna, Airpark Animal Hospital, Westminster, MD
Lindey, Jennifer, Hickory Tree Vet, Winston-Salem, NC
Maedke, Connie, CVT, Animal Hospital of DePere, DePere, WI
Marshall, Danielle, Healthy Pets of Wedgewood, Powell, OH
Mattek, Julie A., CVT, Animal Hospital of Ashwaubenon, Green Bay, WI
Mauldin, Melissa, East Orlando Animal Hospital, Orlando, FL
McCumber, Tiffany, CVT, FIRST Regional Animal Hospital, Chandler, AZ
McFadden, Kathryn, DVM, Towne South Animal Hospital, Shreveport, LA
McIntyre, Jane, Fairway Animal Hospital, Fairway, KS
McPherson, Mary, Animal Health Clinic of Funkstown, Funkstown, MD
Miller, Robin, Suffield Veterinary Hospital, Suffield, CT
Mooney, Allegra, Maple Run Veterinary Clinic LLC, Mount Gilead, OH
Morgan, Cindy, University Hills Animal Hospital, Denver, CO
Morozov, Margaret, Animal Hospital of Sussex County, Augusta, NJ
Morris, Kathy, Elizabeth Animal Hospital, Elizabeth, CO
Neuner, Nicole, McKinney Animal Hospital, McKinney, TX
Nichols, Geri L., LVT, Elliott Bay Animal Hospital, Seattle, WA
Nix, Tiffany, Veterinary Services, Aiken, SC
Noll, Lori, Noll Veterinary Hospital, Springfield, OH

LIST OF CONTRIBUTORS

Nowery, Elaine R., Animal Clinic of Westerville, Inc., Westerville, OH
Pernot, Nikki, McFarland Animal Hospital, McFarland, WI
Peters, Joan, RVT, Kimberly Crest Veterinary Hospital, Davenport, IA
Pfeiff, Susan, CVPM, University Animal Hospital, Tempe, AZ
Racz, Erica, Parkview Veterinary Hospital, Monterey, CA
Ragsdale, Darcie and Laura Ruffner, Golden Triangle Animal Hospital, Southlake, TX
Roebuck, Kim, Great Bridge & Sajo Farm Veterinary Hospitals, Chesapeake & Virginia Beach, VA
Rossi, Stacie K., CVT, Coral Springs Animal Hospital, Coral Springs, FL
Roy, Arlene, CVT, Countryside Veterinary Hospital, LLC, Shelton, CT
Rue, Steven M., Arrowhead Animal Hospital, PC, Westminster, CO
Russell, Catherine, Best Care Pet Hospital, Omaha, NE
Rutz, Melanie, Burlington Veterinary Center, Burlington, CT
Rydzinski, Amy, Evans Animal Hospital, Evans, GA
Sapp, Carol A., CVPM, Maple Tree Veterinary Hospital, Waynesville, NC
Schaperjahn, David, Burnt Hills Veterinary Hospital, Burnt Hills, NY
Schumacher, Chris, Cedarburg Veterinary Clinic, Cedarburg, WI
Selke, Bonnie, LVT, Guilderland Animal Hospital, Altamont, NY
Sharp, Denise, Olney–Sandy Spring Veterinary Hospital, Sandy Spring, MD
Sheats Hodyka, Jodi, Ann Arbor Animal Hospital, Ann Arbor, MI
Shirley, Angie, BLS, Valparaiso, IN
Simon, Cynthia, Griffith Animal Hospitals, Austin, TX
Smith, Donna, LVT, Miller Place Animal Hospital, Miller Place, NY
Smith, Kris, CVPM, Valley Animal Hospital & Pet Resort, Huntsville, AL
Smith, Michele, Merrimac Valley Animal Hospital, Amesbury, MA
Snyder, Lorenzo, CVT, Best Friends Animal Hospital, Billings, MT
Somers, Dennis, DVM, Best Care Pet Hospital, Sioux Falls, SD
Speas, Jessica, Crescenta Canada Pet Hospital, La Crescenta, CA

LIST OF CONTRIBUTORS

Stilwell, Denise, CVT, College Park Road Veterinary Clinic, Ladson, SC
Story, Jennifer, Country Clinic, Toney, AL
Sullivan, Sarah, CVT, Animal Health Center, Watertown, WI
Sunseri, Alice, Angels Camp Veterinary Hospital, Angels Camp, CA
Sutton, Kathryn, CVT, Superior Animal Hospital & Boarding Suites, LTD, Superior, WI
Tassava, Brenda, CVPM, Broad Ripple Animal Clinic, Indianapolis, IN
Taylor, Danylle, Emerald Valley Pet Medical Center, Eugene, OR
Taylor, Joan, LVT, Sheridan Animal Hospital, Buffalo, NY
Thiessen, Laure, Albany County Veterinary Hospital, Albany, NY
Toale, Cyndi, Beneva Animal Hospital, Sarasota, FL
Trunzo, Nicholas, Arden Animal Hospital, Sacramento, CA
Upchurch, Bryan, Animal Clinic of Nassau County, Callahan, FL
Van Harn, Michelle, Animal Emergency Hospital, Grand Rapids, MI
Warner, Vikky, Magrane Pet Medical Center, Mishawaka, IN
Webber, Christine A., Southeast Veterinary Oncology, Orange Park, FL
Wehmeyer, Bridget E., CVT, Riverview Animal Hospital, Durango, CO
Wells, Elizabeth, New Hartford Animal Hospital, Washington Mills, NY
Wilkinson, Sharon, CVT, NorthPaws Veterinary Center, Greenville, RI
Yoakem, Jeremy, Chillicothe Animal Clinic, Chillicothe, OH
Zimmerman, Kristen, Bogue Animal Hospital, Wichita, KS

Note: These names were copied directly from the responses provided, although obvious errors in city or state names and hospitals have been corrected and entries have been edited for consistency. Contributors who preferred to remain anonymous are not listed here. Because the majority of respondents did not include their titles, all titles have been removed for the sake of consistency.

ABOUT THE AUTHOR

For more than 25 years, James E. Guenther, DVM, MBA, MHA, CVPM, AVA, was an equine and companion animal practitioner and owner of a successful veterinary practice in Asheville, North Carolina. During those years, he learned how important business skills are to running a veterinary practice and began to hone his skills as a practice manager, which led him to pursue a dual master's program in Business Administration and Health Administration. The business knowledge he acquired through these courses led him to develop a 24/7 critical care practice in Asheville. At the same time, he became the practice's first hospital administrator.

Dr. Guenther is currently a consultant and one of the principals in Strategic Veterinary Consulting, Inc., in Asheville. He performs practice valuations and financial reviews, and helps practices with management issues, with a special focus on inventory control.

RECOMMENDED READING

AAHA Press offers high-quality, easy-to-use practice management resources for practice owners and managers. Order online at press.aaha.org or call 800-883-6301.

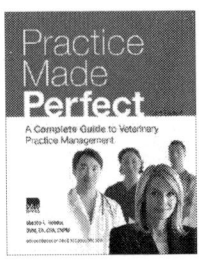

Practice Made Perfect: A Complete Guide to Veterinary Practice Management, Second Edition
Marsha L. Heinke, DVM, EA, CPA, CVPM
Increase your confidence as a manager, ensure financial growth, and foster a team environment in your practice with this bestselling bible of practice management. An excellent resource for any level, this book is required reading for anyone seeking Veterinary Hospital Managers Association certification (VHMA-CVPM).

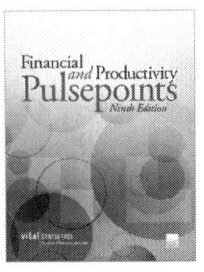

Financial and Productivity Pulsepoints, Ninth Edition
This perennial bestseller offers sound advice—backed by solid data collected from hundreds of hospitals across the country. *Pulsepoints* delivers the measurements, insights, and tools you need to take the competitive edge and run your business brilliantly. The companion website includes benchmarking tools, simulators, a five-episode podcast series on key performance indicators, and more.

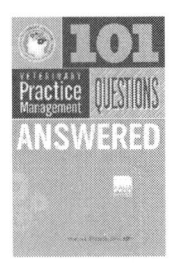

101 Veterinary Practice Management Questions Answered
Amanda L. Donnelly, DVM, MBA
Managers like you pose their most pressing questions, and experts answer them. The handy reference is filled with smart, practical ideas and suggestions.

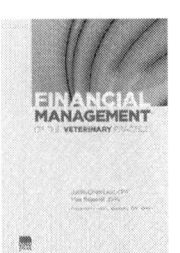

Financial Management of the Veterinary Practice
Justin Chamblee, CPA, MAcc, and Max Reiboldt, CPA
Easy to understand and full of examples, *Financial Management of the Veterinary Practice* will help you establish sound operational processes, make informed decisions, and obtain financial stability.